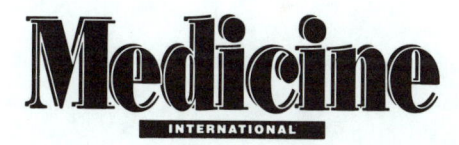

Multiple Choice Questions
Based on the Monthly Add-On Journal

Medicine
INTERNATIONAL

Multiple Choice Questions
Based on the Monthly Add-On Journal

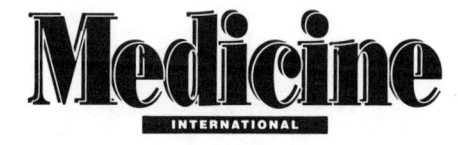

Medicine
INTERNATIONAL

Prepared by Richard L Hawkins MBBS FRCS

PASTEST
Knutsford
Cheshire

© 1995 PASTEST
Egerton Court, Parkgate Estate
Knutsford, Cheshire WA16 8DX
Telephone: 0565 755226

All rights reserved. No part of this publication may be reproduced, stored in a retrieval system, or transmitted, in any form or by any means, electronic, mechanical, photocopying, recording or otherwise without the prior permission of the copyright owner.

First published 1995

ISBN: 0 906896 878

A catalogue record for this book is available from the British Library.

Text prepared by Turner Associates, Knutsford, Cheshire.
Printed and bound in Great Britain by The Cromwell Press, Melksham, Wiltshire.

CONTENTS

Foreword
Introduction
Examination Technique

1.	ALCOHOL/DRUG MISUSE	1
2.	CARDIOLOGY	3
3.	CLINICAL PHARMACOLOGY	12
4.	CRITICAL CARE	18
5.	DERMATOLOGY	20
6.	DIABETES	24
7.	ENDOCRINE DISORDERS	26
8.	GASTROENTEROLOGY	30
9.	GENETICS	38
10.	HAEMATOLOGY	40
11.	IMMUNOLOGY AND AIDS	44
12.	INFECTIONS	48
13.	LIVER DISEASE	56
14.	MULTISYSTEM DISORDERS	60
15.	NEUROLOGY	61
16.	NUTRITION	67
17.	ONCOLOGY	69
18.	ORAL MEDICINE	75
19.	POISONING	76
20.	PSYCHIATRY	78
21.	RENAL DISORDERS	82
22.	RESPIRATORY DISORDERS	88
23.	RHEUMATOLOGY	96
24.	SEXUALLY TRANSMITTED DISEASES	100
	ANSWERS AND TEACHING NOTES	104

FOREWORD

MEDICINE International, the monthly add-on journal, has been published in the UK since 1972. The worldwide readership of the English language editions of the journal approaches 250,000 copies per month, with a distribution covering 110 countries.

Multiple choice questions related to the content of the journal have appeared regularly since the beginning of the first series as an integral part of the journal. In addition, a number of booklets have been published containing further questions relating to the journal. These booklets have been well received because they provide a painless and convenient method for the reader to test his knowledge of the content of the journal and especially, because they closely parallel the kind of questions which appear in so many examinations - especially postgraduate diplomas such as the MRCP, MRCGP and their equivalents around the world.

Over the years, we have made determined efforts to maintain the high quality of the multiple choice questions in the journal. Our collaboration with PasTest has enabled us to produce questions of a consistently high standard. This fourth book contains a large selection of questions on all aspects of clinical internal medicine.

We hope that readers worldwide will find this book of value.

Margaret Stearn MRCP
Medical Editor
MEDICINE International.

INTRODUCTION

The aim of this book is to help the busy doctor test his medical knowledge in his occassional free moments or, if he is working for examinations, to enable him to revise in a methodical manner.

Systematic use of the book should indicate to the reader the subject areas in which he would benefit from further study.

HOW TO USE THIS BOOK

The book can be used on its own as there are brief explanations of the correct answers to all the questions. You will however, obtain far more benefit from the book if you use it in association with MEDICINE International.

Each question is referenced to a particular issue and international page number in all editions of the most recent articles of MEDICINE International. These references are to be found in the answer section of this book from page 99 onwards.

Your method of use of this book will depend on your educational needs and your personal preference. The questions can, of course, be used before and/or after reading the appropriate sections in the journal and many readers find it helpful to 'pre-test' themseleves before deciding upon necessary reading, subsequently 'post-testing' themselves.

Individual study:

- Do not attempt too many questions at one sitting - in this way you are more likely to retain the new knowledge acquired.

- Limit yourself to one group of questions dealing with a specific topic - this should help you to discover your weak points and enable you to use MEDICINE International to revise them.

- Try to avoid looking at the answers before making a definite decision with supporting arguments.

Group discussions:

This can be an effective way to use the book. Ask all participants to test themselves in advance on a set of self-assessment questions and to study their

Introduction

answers in conjunction with the appropriate issues of MEDICINE International. Then discuss the answers with the other members of the group and make further reference to the journal if necessary.

MEDICINE International: you will get maximum value from these questions if you subscribe to MEDICINE International and read each issue as you receive it. The journal contains additional questions, not published in this book, relating to new material as it is published.

PASTEST: if you are working for examinations, other PasTest publications may be of great value to you. There are revision books and/or practice exams available for those preparing for MRCP I & II, MRCGP, MRCOG, DRCOG, DCH, FRCS, FRCA and PLAB.

EXAMINATION TECHNIQUE

The multiple choice questions found in this book are based on the format used in many postgraduate examinations such as the MRCP I, MRCGP, MRCOG, FRCS etc. Each question consists of an initial statement (or 'stem') followed by five possible completions (or 'items') identified by A, B, C, D, E. There is no restriction on the number of true or false items in a question. It is possible for all items in a question to be true or for all to be false.

The four most important points of technique are:

(1) Read the question carefully and be sure you understand it.
(2) Mark your response clearly, correctly and accurately.
(3) Use reasoning to work out answers, but if you do not know the answer and cannot work it out, indicate 'Don't Know'.
(4) The best possible way to obtain a good mark is to have as wide a knowledge as possible of the topics being tested in the examination.

To get the best value from this book you should arrive at an answer either 'True' or 'False' or 'Don't Know' for each item. Commit yourself before you look at the answer - this is really the best way to test your knowledge. In practice you can use the letters 'T', 'F' or 'D' to mark your answer against the question in the book. Alternatively you can prepare a grid on a separate piece of paper thus:-

	A	B	C	D	E
23					
24					

You can then mark your answers on the grid as you go along. To calculate your score give yourself (+1) for each correct item, (-1) for each incorrect item and zero for each 'Don't Know' answer.

All too often examination candidates' marks suffer through an inability to organise their time or through failure to read the instructions carefully. You must ruthlessly allocate your time. For example: in MRCP Part I there are 60 questions to complete in 2 ½ hours, that is 2 ½ minutes per question or 10 questions in 25 minutes. Make sure that you are getting through the exam at this pace or a little quicker to allow time at the end for revision and a re-think on some questions you found difficult.

You must read the question (both stem and items) carefully. You should be quite clear that you know what you are being asked to do. Once you know this, you should indicate your responses by marking the paper boldly, correctly and clearly. In an official examination take great care not to mark the wrong boxes and think very carefully before making a mark on the computer answer sheet. Regard each item as being independent of every other item - each refers to a specific quantum of knowledge. The item (or the stem and the item taken together) make up a statement.

You are required to indicate whether you regard this statement as 'True' or 'False' and you are also able to indicate 'Don't Know'. Look only at a single statement when answering - disregard all the other statements presented in the question, they have nothing to do with the item you are concentrating on.

Since the answer sheets will be read by a computer they must be filled out in accordance with the instructions. As you go through the questions you can either mark your answers immediately on the answer sheet or mark them in the question book in the first instance, transferring them to the answer sheets at the end. In view of the time pressure you may be best advised to mark your answers on the answer sheets as you go along. Don't worry about marking the answer sheet very neatly the first time. Try to leave time to go over your answers again before the end, in particular going back over any difficult questions which you should have marked clearly in your question book. At the same time you can check that you have marked the answer sheet correctly.

Candidates are frequently uncertain whether or not to guess the answer. Experience shows that you should back your 'hunches'. Only if you are completely in the dark should you record a 'Don't Know' answer. Thus, if the question gives you a clue or your knowledge is sufficient to give you a 'hunch' about the correct answer, you will probably gain from guessing.

The answers and explanations in this book are necessarily brief, but they do provide a useful form of revision. The MEDICINE International references with each question give all the background information required to answer that question correctly.

1. ALCOHOL/DRUG MISUSE

1.1 Alcohol dependence syndrome is characterized by

   A poor tolerance for alcohol
   B withdrawal symptoms no longer helped by further drinking
   C no objective or subjective awareness of the compulsion to drink
   D reinstatement after abstinence
   E broadening of drinking repertoire

1.2 The following statements about alcohol are true:

   A per capita alcohol consumption has risen in the last decade in Italy and France
   B a mother would not harm her fetus if she had one or two alcoholic drinks a week
   C in most countries men drink twice as much alcohol as women
   D teenagers who are heavy drinkers have an increased rate of later involvement with illicit drugs
   E currently, alcohol, tobacco and prescribed drugs create more health problems than illicit drug use

1.3 The risk of dying from liver cirrhosis is higher than average in the following groups:

   A farm workers
   B journalists
   C medical practitioners
   D printing machine minders
   E managers in the building and contracting trade

1.4 Ethanol

   A depresses medullary function if drunk excessively
   B has CNS effects directly proportional to the blood ethanol concentration
   C is a peripheral vasoconstrictor
   D inhibits hepatic gluconeogenesis
   E may cause lactic acidosis

1.5 Alcohol withdrawal

A takes a similar clinical course in the vast majority of people
B is characterized by sympathetic nervous system hyperactivity
C may cause hypertension
D is often characterized by inhibition of glucocorticoid secretion
E is frequently complicated by dysrhythmias

1.6 Cannabis

A is usually smoked but can be ingested or injected intravenously
B usually causes bradycardia
C injections produce severe constipation
D use over many years may impair academic performance, which is reversible on cessation of use
E smoke may be carcinogenic

1.7 Volatile substance abuse

A may involve butane and propane
B occurs at some point in about 5% of 15-year-old children in the UK
C in most children lasts less than 6 months
D is more common among girls than boys
E can cause renal failure

2. CARDIOLOGY

2.1 Following myocardial infarction

    A 50% of deaths occur within two hours of onset of symptoms
    B ventricular fibrillation is most likely to occur at 48-72 hours
    C the ECG can remain normal for several hours
    D the ECG can remain normal for several days
    E thrombolytic therapy is contraindicated until chest pain has resolved

2.2 Ejection systolic murmurs may be due to

    A aortic regurgitation
    B pulmonary stenosis
    C atrial septal defects
    D mitral regurgitation
    E aortic sclerosis

2.3 The following conditions are linked together:

    A thyrotoxicosis and rapid ventricular fibrillation
    B Turner's syndrome and coarctation of the aorta
    C myxoedema and cardiomyopathy
    D Down's syndrome and aortic incompetence
    E Marfan's syndrome and patent ductus arteriosus

2.4 Common causes of cardiomegaly include

    A acute myocardial infarction
    B mitral stenosis
    C hypertrophic obstructive cardiomyopathy
    D tricuspid regurgitation
    E aortic regurgitation

2. Cardiology

2.5 The ECG T wave

    A may be inverted in V3 as a normal variant in black people
    B if inverted in V1-V3 in a patient with chest pain, suggests myocardial infarction
    C if generally flattened suggests hypokalaemia
    D if found in the anterior leads may suggest hypertrophic cardiomyopathy
    E if associated with downward sloping ST, suggests drug effect

2.6 The following statements about cardiac catheterization are true:

    A the left atrium is the chamber most easily entered
    B pressure in the left ventricle is usually measured by advancing a catheter through the femoral or antecubital vein
    C direct left atrial catheterization can sometimes be performed through a patent foramen ovale
    D cine angiography is a reliable way of detecting ventricular aneurysms
    E a gradient of 30 mm Hg across the aortic valve indicates severe stenosis

2.7 Factors predisposing to palpitations include

    A alcohol
    B gastro-oesophageal reflux
    C methyldopa
    D Parkinson's disease
    E sympathomimetic drugs

2.8 The following drugs may cause bradycardia:

    A aminophylline
    B lithium
    C digoxin
    D verapamil
    E bethanidine

2. Cardiology

2.9 The immediate management of acute heart failure should include

- A putting the patient in a supine position to reduce the work-load on the heart
- B avoiding morphine because it sedates the patient
- C administering frusemide for its vasodilating effect as well as diuretic effect
- D administering digoxin for its positive inotropic effect on the heart
- E avoiding nitrates which have a negative inotropic effect on the heart

2.10 Vasodilators in patients with heart failure

- A increase cardiac output
- B increase left atrial pressure
- C reduce the venous filling pressure of the ventricles
- D are particularly valuable for long term treatment
- E lower systemic vascular resistance

2.11 Angiotensin converting enzyme inhibitors

- A reduce renal perfusion
- B should not be used with potassium sparing diuretics
- C increase venous pressure
- D increase blood flow to exercising skeletal tissue
- E are contraindicated in the presence of severe heart failure

2.12 Dilated cardiomyopathy

- A is usually accompanied by hypertension
- B is often complicated by supraventricular and ventricular arrhythmias
- C is a contraindication to coronary arteriography
- D should be treated by calcium antagonists as first-line therapy
- E should be treated by anti-coagulation if there is evidence of moderate left ventricular dilatation

2. Cardiology

2.13 The following statements about left venticular aneurysms are true:

A the anterior or apical segment of the ventricle is the most common site for an aneurysm
B most aneurysms are due to occlusion of the right coronary artery
C the 5-year survival rate varies between 60% and 75%
D systemic emboli from the ventricular wall occur in over 50% of cases
E congestive heart failure is a contraindication to surgery

2.14 Recognized clinical features of rupture of interventricular septum include

A the development of a new diastolic murmur
B systemic hypotension
C raised jugular venous pressure
D the development of a new cardiac thrill
E palpitations

2.15 A high mortality following myocardial infarction is associated with

A increasing age
B high blood pressure
C high heart rate on admission to hospital
D anterior infarction pattern on ECG
E previous infarction

2.16 Nitrates

A cause venous constriction
B increase venous return
C increase cardiac output
D generally give relief from angina for no longer than 10 minutes
E are not subject to first-pass metabolism in the liver

2. Cardiology

2.17 Angioplasty

- A is ideal for treatment of a discrete stenosis of the main stem of the left coronary artery
- B is dangerous for patients with multiple vessel disease
- C is contraindicated in patients who have undergone bypass surgery
- D is contraindicated in patients with unstable angina
- E usually involves complications if there is acute occlusion of the lesion

2.18 Complications following coronary angiography

- A include a mortality rate of about 5%
- B include a myocardial infarction rate of about 0.2%
- C include a thromboembolic stroke rate of about 0.1%
- D increase with the severity of the patient's symptoms
- E occur at the arterial entry site in about 0.1% of procedures

2.19 Following myocardial infarction the chances of recurrence can be reduced if

- A the patient stops smoking
- B the patient is routinely started on an anti-arrhythmic drug
- C the patient is started on a β-blocker
- D the patient is started on daily low-dose aspirin
- E the patient is started on a low cholesterol diet

2.20 The following statements about cardiac enzymes are true:

- A cardiac enzymes are produced by normal heart cells to repair heart cells damaged by infarction
- B the level of lactic dehydrogenase activity is the first enzymatic level to rise following myocardial infarction
- C the profile of creatine kinase activity is altered by early reperfusion of infarcted myocardium
- D peak lactic dehydrogenase activity gives a crude estimate of myocardial infarction size
- E raised plasma creatine kinase levels can result from skeletal as well as cardiac muscle damage

2. Cardiology

2.21 Concordance of blood pressure levels can be shown between

    A siblings
    B non-identical twins
    C parents and children
    D parents and adopted children
    E husbands and wives

2.22 In intermittent claudication

    A the clinical course is more benign in women than in men
    B the measurement of the resting arm:thigh Doppler pressure index is a valuable investigation
    C most patients' symptoms steadily deteriorate following presentation
    D life expectancy is shorter than in unaffected individuals
    E regular exercise improves blood flow in the long term

2.23 The following statements about hypertension are true:

    A if postural hypotension is suspected, blood pressure measurement should be taken in the supine position
    B in pregnant women, blood pressure measurement should be taken in the supine position
    C pressure readings may be artificially low in obese individuals if standard sized cuffs are used
    D a pressure difference of more than 5 mm Hg between the two arms of a patient is pathological
    E most patients show a defence reaction with artificially raised blood pressure

2.24 The following drugs should be avoided in hypertensive patients with the following conditions:

    A thiazide diuretics in patients with gout
    B calcium antagonists in patients with glucose intolerance
    C β-blockers in patients with cardiac failure
    D calcium antagonists in patients with ischaemic heart disease
    E β-blockers in patients with obstructive airways disease

2. Cardiology

2.25 Percutaneous transluminal femoral angioplasty

    A can be performed under local anaesthesia
    B has a success rate of about 50%
    C should not be repeated more than once at the same site
    D can be combined with local fibrinolytic therapy
    E has a mortality of 10%

2.26 The signs of pericardial effusion include

    A reduced cardiac dullness on percussion
    B an easily palpable apex beat
    C low pulse pressure
    D pulsus paradoxus
    E raised jugular venous pressure

2.27 In acute pericarditis

    A chest auscultation may reveal a presystolic friction rub
    B the ECG characteristically shows depressed ST segments
    C the chest radiograph characteristically shows patchy areas of consolidation
    D a normal echocardiogram does not exclude the diagnosis
    E the ESR is normally raised

2.28 The following statements about blood pressure are true:

    A blood pressure rises in the first few weeks of life
    B blood pressure among post-menopausal females is usually higher than similarly aged males
    C there is no relation between an individual's blood pressure at an early age and in old age
    D blood pressure is lower in those who exercise regularly than in those who do not
    E alcohol consumption has minimal impact upon blood pressure

2.29 Children with tetralogy of Fallot

A present with an ejection diastolic murmur
B are prone to hypoxic spells
C may have an absent pulmonary second sound if the condition is severe
D may be treated by a Blalock shunt
E often squat during exercise as this produces the beneficial effect of reducing systemic resistance by compressing the femoral arteries

2.30 Central cyanosis

A occurs when the concentration of reduced haemoglobin in the blood exceeds 5 g/dl
B is more apparent in anaemic children than in those with normal haemoglobin levels
C occurs when venous blood by-passes the lungs
D is often characterized in babies by the appearance of finger clubbing within days of birth
E may occur due to a severe ventricular septal defect

2.31 Large ventricular septal defects

A are well tolerated by most infants
B can cause pulmonary hypertension
C usually present towards the end of the first month of life
D can cause congestive heart failure
E are surgically treated by direct repair of the septal defect

2.32 Coarctation of the aorta in neonates

A should be investigated by cardiac catheterization in most cases
B is associated with upper body hypertension
C causes low pulmonary pressure
D may be improved by re-opening the ductus arteriosus
E may need treatment with catecholamines

2. Cardiology

2.33 The signs of aortic regurgitation include

    A visible capillary pulsation in the fingers
    B head bobbing
    C early diastolic murmur
    D a loud aortic second sound
    E hepatomegaly

2.34 The causes of mitral regurgitation include

    A rheumatoid arthritis
    B left atrial myxoma
    C atrial septal defect
    D ventricular septal defect
    E Marfan's syndrome

2.35 The indications for aortic valvotomy in the treatment of congenital aortic stenosis include

    A ECG changes of right ventricular hypertrophy
    B minimal pressure drop across the aortic valve
    C total fusion of two valve cusps
    D significant risk of sudden death
    E ECG changes of left ventricular hypertrophy

3. CLINICAL PHARMACOLOGY

3.1 **Drug metabolism**

    A occurs mainly in the liver
    B usually requires two separate phases - oxidation and conjugation
    C is impaired in premature babies
    D occurs more rapidly in full-term babies and children than in adults
    E is slower in those who smoke than in those who do not

3.2 **Drug absorption**

    A occurs predominantly in the stomach
    B is slowed by opiates
    C is quicker for lipid soluble drugs than for water soluble drugs
    D is best achieved by water soluble drugs in the presence of food
    E is slowed by extensive gastrointestinal disease, water soluble drugs being more affected than lipid soluble ones

3.3 **The following statements about drugs are true:**

    A peak drug concentrations are usually reached 10-20 minutes following ingestion
    B the oral route of administration of a drug is invariably the safest route
    C enteric coated aspirin does not have an irritant effect on the gastric mucosa
    D slow-release formulations are designed for drugs with a long elimination half-life
    E the purpose of sublingual administration is to bypass the problems of gastric absorption

3.4 **The indications for measuring serum drug concentration include**

    A drugs whose serum concentration and therapeutic effect are difficult to relate
    B drugs which have a narrow therapeutic range
    C drugs which have an immediate response which is easy to assess
    D occasions when the initial prescription of a drug has proved ineffective
    E suspected pharmacokinetic drug interactions

3. Clinical Pharmacology

3.5 The following receptors and antagonists are linked:

A histamine receptors and methysergide
B adrenoreceptors and practolol
C 5-HT receptors and cimetidine
D dopamine receptors and phenothiazines
E cholinoceptors and atropine

3.6 The following drugs are enzyme inducers:

A phenobarbitone
B oral contraceptives
C cimetidine
D phenytoin
E rifampicin

3.7 The following drugs are enzyme inhibitors:

A ethanol (chronic)
B carbemazepine
C sulphinpyrazone
D chlorpromazine
E erythromycin

3.8 The following statements about the elderly are true:

A glomerular filtration rate increases by 50% between 50 and 90 years of age
B there is a 40% decline in liver blood flow between 40 and 80 years of age
C the proportion of slow acetylators is higher in people over 65 years than in those under 65 years
D the relative increase in body fat in people over 65 years lengthens the elimination half-life of lipophilic drugs
E enzyme induction is blunted in old age

3. Clinical Pharmacology

3.9 Glucocorticoids

A depress neutrophil function
B significantly raise blood levels of IgE
C may cause hypokalaemia at high doses
D often cause a growth spurt in children
E are linked with osteopetrosis

3.10 Calcium-channel blockers

A are contraindicated in patients with angina
B stimulate the uptake of calcium into cardiac cells
C are contraindicated in chronic obstructive lung disease
D reduce myocardial blood flow
E cause coronary artery vasodilation

3.11 Recognized side-effects of theophylline include

A muscle tremor
B hypokalaemia
C convulsions
D impaired learning ability in children
E acute hypertension

3.12 The following statements about antithrombotic drugs are true:

A warfarin inhibits the synthesis of biologically active plasminogen
B heparin stimulates the synthesis of biologically active prothrombin
C one of the actions of dextran is to interfere with platelet function
D streptokinase is extracted from β-haemolytic streptococci
E APSAC has been designed to bind selectively to fibrin

3. Clinical Pharmacology

3.13 The taking of oral contraceptive steroids makes a woman more susceptible to

   A benign breast disease
   B carcinoma of the ovary
   C venous thrombosis
   D carcinoma of the uterus
   E pancreatitis

3.14 The following drugs are suitable for breast-feeding women:

   A sulphonamides
   B aspirin
   C lithium
   D cephalosporins
   E tricyclic antidepressants

3.15 The following drugs and adverse reactions are linked:

   A clindamycin and retroperitoneal fibrosis
   B metoclopromide and aplastic anaemia
   C phenylbutazone and aplastic anaemia
   D chloramphenicol and acute dystonia
   E methysergide and pseudomembranous colitis

3.16 Adverse drug reactions

   A are responsible for about 4% of all hospital admissions
   B occur in 10-20% of hospital in-patients
   C occur more commonly in women than in men
   D occur more commonly in atopic patients than those with no history of atopy
   E occur more commonly in certain ethnic groups than in others

3. Clinical Pharmacology

3.17 **The following statements about drugs are true:**

A generally drugs are absorbed from the small bowel rather than from the stomach
B malabsorption syndromes have a profound effect on the absorption of most drugs
C the liver is the most important site of first-pass metabolism
D for most drugs the clearance, volume of distribution and half-life are the same at different doses
E the half-life, rather than the rate of clearance of a drug, is the best measure of the rate at which a drug is eliminated from the body

3.18 **The following statements about routes of drug administration are true:**

A sublingual administration of the drug by-passes first-pass degradation by the liver
B subcutaneous absorption of drugs is faster than intramuscular absorption
C low molecular weight drugs, soluble in both oil and water, are suitable for transdermal administration
D the bioavailability of drugs undergoing marked first-pass liver metabolism is increased by simultaneous food intake
E the transit time of the oesophagus by a tablet is unaffected by lying supine

3.19 **The following drugs may be effectively administered rectally:**

A morphine
B diazepam
C sodium valproate
D paracetamol
E indomethacin

3. Clinical Pharmacology

3.20 The bioavailability of the following drugs is increased by the concurrent intake of food:

    A ampicillin
    B captopril
    C tetracycline
    D chloroquine
    E propranolol

3.21 The following drugs have the following modes of action:

    A atenolol is a β-receptor agonist
    B minoxidil is a calcium channel blocker
    C lignocaine is a sodium channel blocker
    D allopurinol is a xanthine oxidase inhibitor
    E nifedipine is a potassium channel opener

3.22 Routine therapeutic drug monitoring is advisable for the following drugs:

    A ethosuximide
    B lithium
    C sodium valproate
    D primidone
    E phenytoin

3.23 The following drugs are linked with the following adverse reactions:

    A stilboestrol with jaundice
    B halothane with pulmonary embolism
    C isoprenaline with acute dystonia
    D phenylbutazone with aplastic anaemia
    E chloramphenicol with pseudo-membranous colitis

4. CRITICAL CARE

4.1 Mechanical ventilation

A aims at an inspiratory:expiratory ratio of 1:2 for most patients
B lowers cardiac output
C increases the risk of pneumothorax
D is advantageous for left ventricular failure
E predisposes to right heart failure in asthmatics

4.2 In the management of patients with life-threatening sepsis

A antibiotics should be withheld until the focus of infection has been identified
B prophylaxis against *Candida* spp should be routinely administered
C sucralfate has a useful role in maintaining gastrointestinal perfusion
D corticosteroids should be routinely given
E dopamine improves renal blood flow, particularly in the presence of vasoconstrictor inotropes

4.3 The following conditions predispose to sepsis:

A alcoholism
B uraemia
C obesity
D antacid therapy
E nasotracheal tubes

4.4 The following conditions are associated with adult respiratory distress syndrome:

A pre-eclampsia
B pancreatitis
C raised intracranial pressure
D asthma
E oxygen toxicity

4. Critical Care

4.5 Morphine

- A increases gastrointestinal motility
- B uptake by the CNS is potentiated by acidaemia
- C can cause truncal rigidity
- D has an elimination half-life which is reduced in patients with impaired liver function
- E has a prolonged ventilatory depressive effect in patients with impaired renal function

4.6 The following statements about the management of drowning are correct:

- A active core warming is needed if the patient's core temperature is below 32 °C
- B anti-arrhythmics should be used routinely despite their myocardial depressant effect
- C barbiturates provide useful neuronal protection
- D corticosteroids provide protection against wet lung syndrome
- E 'rewarming shock' is treated by increasing intravenous fluids

4.7 Ventricular fibrillation

- A is the most likely arrhythmia in the early stages of a cardiac arrest
- B should be treated by immediate AC cardioversion
- C if refractory, should be treated by increasing levels of cardioversion energy to a maximum of 3200 J
- D if refractory, can be successfully treated by a bolus of bretylium tosylate
- E if refractory, should be treated with adrenaline before giving lignocaine

4.8 The following drugs are appropriate for the treatment of ventricular tachycardia:

- A dopamine
- B bretylium
- C lignocaine
- D mysoline
- E disopyramide

5. DERMATOLOGY

5.1 The following dermatological terms are accurately described:

- A cicatrice is a horny thickening of the skin
- B papule is a non-palpable, discoloured area of skin up to 1 cm in diameter
- C erythema is redness of the skin which does not blanche on pressure
- D acanthosis is thickening of the prickle cell layer of the epidermis
- E bulla is a fluid-filled elevation of skin greater than 0.5 cm in diameter

5.2 The following drugs may precipitate or exacerbate psoriasis:

- A lithium
- B hydralazine
- C H_2-antagonists
- D β-blockers
- E anticonvulsants

5.3 The following drugs are characteristically linked with the following type of reaction:

- A oral contraceptives and photosensitivity
- B codeine and urticaria
- C tetracycline and exfoliative dermatitis
- D fucidin and pigmentation
- E β-blockers and eczema

5.4 The following conditions are associated with erythema nodosum:

- A herpes simplex
- B tuberculosis
- C inflammatory bowel disease
- D hyperthyroidism
- E Behçet's syndrome

5. Dermatology

5.5 The following skin conditions generally deteriorate during pregnancy:

- A atopic eczema
- B systemic lupus erythematosus
- C candidiasis
- D hidradenitis suppurativa
- E herpes simplex

5.6 The characteristic skin lesions of tuberous sclerosis include

- A milia
- B mongolian patches
- C port wine stains
- D irregularly coarsened sacral skin (shagreen patch)
- E oval hypopigmented areas (ash leaf macules)

5.7 Atopic dermatitis

- A is synonymous with atopic eczema
- B affects infants on the nappy area most characteristically
- C affects adults characteristically on the extensor surfaces of hands and feet
- D does not develop in infants who are breast fed
- E clears from most affected patients by 13 years of age

5.8 The following facial conditions are linked to the following diagnostic signs:

- A rosacea and pimples sparing the immediate vermillion border
- B erysipelas and a tender, indurated eruption
- C carcinoid syndrome and a vascular, bright red eruption usually lasting a few days at a time
- D dermatomyositis and a violet-red, telangiectatic eruption with a photosensitive distribution
- E superior vena caval obstruction and fixed facial cyanosis, often with distended veins and oedema

5. Dermatology

5.9 Nails with the following signs are suggestive of the following conditions:

A transverse grooves and psoriasis
B opaque nails and diabetes mellitus
C splinter haemorrhages and bacterial endocarditis
D blue nails and *Pseudomonas* spp. infection
E longitudinal ridges and lichen planus

5.10 The following statments about pruritus are true:

A cholestatic pruritus is probably due to an increase of bile salts in the skin
B drugs which slow hepatic microsomal function may improve cholestatic pruritus
C pruritus is a common symptom of diabetes mellitus
D pruritus is a symptom of both hyperthyroidism and hypothyroidism
E pruritus is a recognized symptom of folate deficiency

5.11 The following skin lesions are benign:

A seborrhoeic ketatosis
B lentigine
C large (diameter greater than 5 cm) congenital melanocytic naevi
D dysplastic naevi
E blue naevi

5.12 Basal cell carcinoma

A is the most common skin malignancy in caucasians
B almost never occurs on covered skin sites
C is characterized histologically by cells containing large, poorly staining nuclei and abundant cytoplasm
D should not any longer be treated by curettage and cautery since results are inferior to other treatment methods
E may appear in organoid naevi

5. Dermatology

5.13 Bowen's disease

- A is a multi-system disease of which the skin is an important part
- B involves sun exposed skin sites more than covered sites
- C particularly affects people of African origin
- D is significantly linked with internal malignancy
- E is primarily a tumour of the endodermal skin layer

5.14 Dermatophyte infection

- A rarely causes alopecia
- B can be diagnosed using blue-green fluorescence under ultraviolet light using a Wood's light
- C can be successfully treated by griseofulvin or terbinafine
- D may become malignant if the infection is left untreated and becomes chronic
- E is one of the presenting features of dermatomyositis

5.15 The following statements about acne vulgaris are true:

- A most teenagers with acne seek no treatment for it
- B the key pathological event in acne is obstruction of the pilosebaceous duct
- C the severity of acne is directly related to the degree of secretion of sebum
- D circulating levels of androgen are usually high in patients with acne
- E an open comedo (blackhead) results from the rupture of the wall of the pilosebaceous duct and release of the contents in the dermis

6. DIABETES

6.1 Non-insulin dependent diabetes mellitus

    A is more prevalent than insulin-dependent diabetes mellitus in all populations
    B is a mild form of diabetes mellitus which reduces life expectancy only minimally
    C is seldom accompanied by macrovascular disease
    D is characterized by marked sensitivity to insulin action
    E can be successfully treated by dietary modification alone

6.2 The following statements are good dietary advice for diabetic patients:

    A diabetics will need to eat a specialized diet which is markedly different from the rest of the family
    B diet has an important role in the management of non-insulin dependent diabetes but not insulin dependent diabetes
    C fat should preferably be taken as saturated fat
    D maintaining a low carbohydrate intake is an important aspect of a diabetic diet
    E alcohol should be avoided by patients taking insulin or oral hypoglycaemics because it has a hyperglycaemic effect

6.3 The following features are characteristic of diabetic retinopathy:

    A arterio-venous nipping
    B hard exudates
    C microaneurysms
    D papilloedema
    E new vessel formation

6.4 The following are tests of autonomic function:

    A lying and standing blood pressure
    B Tinel's sign
    C dark adapted pupil diameter
    D Valsalva response
    E plantar reflexes

6. Diabetes

6.5 Diabetic nephropathy

A is responsible for 25% of the deaths in diabetic patients diagnosed before the age of 30 years
B usually causes end-stage renal failure 7-10 years after the appearance of persistent proteinuria
C should be routinely investigated by renal biopsy
D is commonly associated with coronary artery disease
E can be reversed by tight control of blood sugar levels

6.6 In diabetic ketoacidosis

A leucocytosis is common and does not confirm infection
B serum amylase levels may be raised, and it is not due to pancreatitis
C urinary stick testing for ketones may be negative
D plasma glucose may be low
E a normal plasma potassium level excludes significant potassium deficiency

6.7 The following statements about diabetic ketoacidosis are true:

A with treatment there is still an average mortality of 15%
B about 30% of cases occur in patients with previously unrecognized diabetes
C in about 10-15% of cases no identifiable cause is found
D infection is the cause in about half the cases where an identifiable cause is found
E without treatment there is an average mortality of about 50%

7. ENDOCRINE DISORDERS

7.1 The following statements about acromegaly are correct:

    A diagnosis is based on showing that growth hormone levels do not rise normally after an oral glucose load
    B about 75% of patients have impaired glucose tolerance
    C most cases are due to a pituitary tumour
    D the modern definitive treatment is bromocriptine administration
    E hypertension is a well recognized feature

7.2 Graves' disease is distinguished clinically from other forms of hyperthyroidism by

    A diffuse thyroid enlargement over which there may be a bruit
    B proximal myopathy
    C pretibial myxoedema
    D ophthalmopathy
    E gynaecomastia

7.3 Hypothyroidism

    A should be treated with a high replacement dose of T3 initially, gradually reducing over 3 weeks
    B is usually secondary to failure of thyroid stimulating hormone secretion
    C is common in patients with Down's syndrome
    D is common in patients receiving lithium carbonate
    E causes reduction in growth velocity in children

7.4 Papillary thyroid carcinoma

    A is usually unifocal
    B typically spreads to regional lymph nodes
    C is more common among women under 50 years of age
    D has a poor prognosis because metastasis to the lungs is common
    E may be treated by near-total or total thyroidectomy

7. Endocrine Disorders

7.5 Addison's disease

A affects about 0.5% of the British population
B is named after a Boston neurosurgeon
C is characterized by low plasma ACTH
D is diagnosed using the short Guthrie test
E is a contraindication to pregnancy

7.6 Vasopressin

A migrates to the anterior pituitary in neurosecretory granules
B secretion is suppressed when plasma osmolality falls
C acts by making the collecting tubules of the kidneys more permeable to water
D can cause splanchnic vasoconstriction
E stimulates glycogenolysis

7.7 The syndrome of inappropriate antidiuresis may be caused by

A carbamazepine
B thiazide diuretics
C vasopressin
D MAO1 antidepressants
E carbidopa

7.8 Parathyroid hormone

A serum levels cannot be reliably measured
B is synthesised in response to hypercalcaemia
C serves as a trophic hormone to convert 25-hydroxycholecalciferol to 1,25-dihydroxycholecalciferol
D is inhibited by the active metabolite of vitamin D
E can cause osteitis fibrosa cystica

7. Endocrine Disorders

7.9 The causes of delayed puberty include

    A cystic fibrosis
    B sarcoidosis
    C testicular torsion
    D retractile testes
    E Klinefelter's syndrome

7.10 Testosterone

    A stimulates spermatogenesis
    B stimulates Leydig cells in the seminiferous tubules to secrete inhibin
    C has a direct negative feedback effect on gonadotrophin releasing hormone
    D failure in the first trimester of gestation results in pseudohermaphroditism
    E is produced by Sertoli cells of the seminiferous tubules

7.11 Gynaecomastia

    A occurs in 50% of normal boys during puberty
    B commonly occurs in neonates as a result of suckling on mother's milk
    C may occur secondarily to a decline in serum testosterone levels
    D is a recognized feature of Klinefelter's syndrome
    E is a complication of methyldopa

7.12 Classical findings in the polycystic ovary syndrome include

    A lowered serum LH
    B lowered serum prolactin
    C raised serum testosterone
    D raised serum FSH
    E normal serum thyroxine

7. Endocrine Disorders

7.13 **The following facts about the menopause are true:**

A   the menopause is due to loss of pituitary drive to the ovaries
B   up to 10% of cases of postmenopausal bleeding are due to malignancy
C   a premenopausal woman's risk of coronary artery disease is one fifth of that of a man of the same age
D   osteoclastic bone formation is slowed by the menopause
E   postmenopausal women at risk of osteoporosis should be encouraged to take calcium supplements

7.14 **The following facts about endocrine hypertension are true:**

A   endocrine hypertension accounts for about 25% of all cases of hypertension
B   all hypertensive patients should undergo full endocrine screening
C   the WHO definition of definite hypertension is a blood pressure of over 180/105 mm Hg
D   raised serum testosterone is the most common cause of endocrine hypertension in the developed world
E   the progesterone-only pill (or mini-pill) is the contraceptive pill most likely to raise blood pressure

8. GASTROENTEROLOGY

8.1 Duodenal ulceration

A usually occurs in the duodenal bulb
B affects approximately 10% of the population
C has been proved to be caused by non-steroidal anti-inflammatory drugs
D has a natural history of settling spontaneously within 5-10 years of onset
E causes pain with a characteristic history and presentation

8.2 The following statements about benign gastric ulceration are true:

A benign ulceration occurs most commonly on the greater curve of the stomach
B benign ulceration rarely penetrates into the muscularis mucosa
C patients with benign ulcers secrete greater than normal amounts of gastric acid
D benign gastric ulceration affects men and women equally
E a careful history will readily distinguish gastric ulcer pain from duodenal ulcer pain

8.3 The following skin conditions and gastrointestinal diseases are linked:

A erythema nodosum and inflammatory bowel disease
B spider naevi and hepatic disease
C acanthosis nigricans and gastrointestinal malignancy
D mucocutaneous pigmentation and Peutz-Jeghers syndrome
E pyoderma gangrenosum and coeliac disease

8.4 Acute upper gastrointestinal haemorrhage

A has an overall mortality of 1%
B is most commonly caused by bleeding from oesophageal varices
C is strongly associated with steroid therapy
D can be gauged accurately by haemoglobin estimation
E is a complication of overwhelming sepsis

8. Gastroenterology

8.5 **The following statements about gastric adenocarcinoma are true:**

A in Western countries there has been a marked increase in the incidence over the last 50 years
B the tumour is more common in high socio-economic groups than in low socio-economic groups
C the tumour is common in Japan
D once lymph nodes are involved, the 5-year survival is approximately 10%
E radiotherapy has a valuable complementary role to surgery

8.6 **The following factors are associated with an increased risk of gastric adenocarcinoma:**

A high salt intake
B exposure to rubber processing
C living in areas with a low iodine content in the soil
D living in areas with a high nitrate content in the soil
E chronic gastritis

8.7 **Double-contrast barium meal**

A coats the gastric mucosa with a thin layer of concentrated barium and a thicker layer of dilute barium
B requires no prior preparation
C is more operator-dependent than single-contrast barium studies
D often causes diarrhoea
E accurately reveals gastric lesions over 0.5 cm in diameter

8.8 **The following statements about coeliac disease are true:**

A many adults do not have a childhood history
B the symptoms in childhood may improve by adolescence without treatment
C most patients respond to a gluten diet within 1 month
D there is an increased likelihood of oesophageal cancer
E there is an increased risk of pemphigus

8. Gastroenterology

8.9 Lactose intolerance

    A causes osteoporosis due to poor milk intake
    B in its primary form is more common in northern Europeans than in people of African descent
    C is linked with HLA-B8
    D is demonstrated by high levels of lactase in jejunal biopsy
    E can be diagnosed by measuring hydrogen levels in the breath after a lactose load

8.10 The following investigation results occur characteristically in patients with post-infective malabsorption:

    A normal xylose absorption test
    B normal Schilling test
    C increased faecal fat excretion
    D flat villi on jejunal biopsy
    E low serum zinc and magnesium levels

8.11 The complications of cystic fibrosis include

    A heartburn
    B rectal prolapse
    C cirrhosis
    D coagulopathy
    E portal hypertension

8.12 Pancreatic cancer

    A is more common today than 50 years ago
    B has an overall 5-year survival rate of 1%
    C usually occurs as a squamous cell tumour
    D occurs more commonly in the body and tail of the pancreas than in the head
    E can be diagnosed reliably by tumour-specific antigen measurements

8. Gastroenterology

8.13 Acute pancreatitis

A can occur without pain
B is usually due to excessive alcohol intake
C is diagnosed once the serum amylase level is double the upper limit of normal
D may be complicated by acute hypoglycaemia due to excessive insulin secretion
E should never be investigated by ERCP for safety reasons

8.14 Complications of short bowel syndrome include

A kidney stone
B gallstones
C metabolic alkalosis
D hypocalcaemia
E hypoproteinaemia

8.15 Acute appendicitis

A is the most common acute abdominal emergency requiring surgery
B is common in elderly people and in children under 12 years of age
C is almost always associated with a raised WBC
D is usually caused by the bacteria *Escherichia coli*
E can be diagnosed reliably by abdominal radiography

8.16 The following drugs may cause constipation:

A aluminium trisilicate
B tricyclic antidepressants
C oral contraceptives
D cimetidine
E iron

8. Gastroenterology

8.17 Non-colonic features of irritable bowel syndrome include

    A dyspareunia
    B erythema nodosum
    C uveitis
    D arthritis
    E urinary frequency

8.18 Irritable bowel syndrome

    A is more common in women than in men
    B often presents in middle to old age
    C causes abdominal pain made worse by defaecation
    D causes rectal bleeding
    E seldom affects children

8.19 The following features are more characteristic of Crohn's disease than of ulcerative colitis:

    A abdominal mass
    B bloody diarrhoea
    C aphthoid ulcers
    D destruction of mucin glands
    E perianal disease

8.20 The following statements about the aetiology and course of Crohn's disease are true:

    A a high-fibre diet improves the prognosis
    B a low-sugar diet improves the prognosis
    C smokers are more liable to develop Crohn's disease than non-smokers
    D a link with the intestinal organism *Mycobacterium paratuberculosis* has been postulated
    E there is a strong genetic link among Jews

8. Gastroenterology

8.21 The following statements about gastrointestinal histoplasmosis are true:

A it is a protozoal disease caused by *Histoplasma capsulatum*
B it occurs only in North America
C it produces granulomatous lesions which may affect any part of the gastrointestinal tract, from the mouth to the rectum
D it is best diagnosed on complement fixation tests
E treatment is most effective with rifampicin

8.22 The following are recognized complications of stomas:

A dermatitis
B renal calculi
C gallstones
D water overload
E parastomal hernia

8.23 Colonoscopy should be avoided in patients with

A chronic inflammatory bowel disease
B colonic cancer
C profuse rectal bleeding
D ascites
E peritonism

8.24 Colorectal cancer

A is the most common gastrointestinal malignancy in the developed world
B probably arises from benign adenomas
C could be eliminated by effective screening
D can usually be detected by careful abdominal palpation
E has a familial tendency in a small number of cases

8. Gastroenterology

8.25 The following statements about ischaemic bowel disease are true:

A occlusion of the superior mesenteric artery usually results in ischaemia of the sigmoid colon
B the ascending colon is the most vulnerable segment of the colon
C muscle is more sensitive to ischaemia than mucosa
D patients seldom have evidence of vascular disease elsewhere
E angiography is a vital and helpful immediate investigation

8.26 Diverticular disease

A often occurs without symptoms
B affects the transverse colon more commonly than the sigmoid colon
C commonly presents with rectal bleeding
D should not be treated with morphine as it increases muscle spasm
E usually requires immediate surgery

8.27 Primary herpes simplex proctitis in homosexual men

A is usually caused by herpes simplex type 1
B does not usually cause inguinal lymphadenopathy
C may produce neurological symptoms
D can usefully be treated with oral acyclovir
E is more common in those patients who are immunocompromised

8.28 The following advice about meals should be given to patients with late dumping syndrome:

A eat solid food first
B eat meals slowly
C ensure high levels of carbohydrates in the diet
D avoid high fibre food
E adopt the 'Roman' position (lying on the left side) while eating

8. Gastroenterology

8.29 **The following are recognized complications of gastric surgery:**

- A gastric cancer following a polya-type gastrectomy
- B increased incidence of atherosclerosis
- C folate deficiency anaemia
- D osteoporosis
- E cholelithiasis

9. GENETICS

9.1 The following investigations are appropriate for the conditions given:

    A fetal tissue sampling and epidermolysis bullosa
    B chorionic villus sampling and haemoglobinopathies
    C maternal serum α-fetoprotein and cystic fibrosis
    D amniocentesis and Down's syndrome
    E ultrasound and congenital heart disease

9.2 Chromosomes

    A are numbered from the largest (number 1) to the smallest (number 22 in humans)
    B carry many thousands of genes each
    C have a short 'p' arm and a long 'q' arm
    D are abnormal in approximately 0.5% live births
    E are commonly stained to show G-banding

9.3 The following statements are true:

    A most DNA has no known function
    B there are about 5000 genes
    C cloning is the production of identical copies of isolated fragments of DNA
    D the human haploid genome consists of about three billion base pairs of double-stranded DNA
    E DNA is usually fragmented using restriction enzymes

9.4 Duchenne muscular dystrophy

    A is the most common X-linked recessive disease
    B normally restricts affected children to a wheelchair by the age of 12 years
    C is linked with the partial or complete absence of the muscle protein actin
    D affects girls more than boys
    E can be diagnosed using genetic probes

9. Genetics

9.5 **The following facts about Huntington's disease are true:**

    A the children of an individual with Huntington's disease have a 25% chance of developing the disease themselves
    B Huntington's disease affects more males than females
    C new mutations make up approximately 50% of cases
    D there is a tendency for paternal transmission to children to result in earlier onset of the disease
    E the Huntington's disease gene has still not been located to a chromosome

9.6 **The clinical features of Wilson's disease include**

    A peripheral sensory neuropathy
    B psychosis
    C resting tremor
    D Maxwell's ring
    E dysarthria

9.7 **Classical phenylketonuria**

    A is due to an inborn error of renal excretion of phenylalanine
    B is associated with impairment of melanin production
    C is treated by a strict low phenylalanine, low tyrosine diet for life
    D can not be diagnosed prenatally
    E does not harm the fetus of an affected woman

10. HAEMATOLOGY

10.1 The following statements about laboratory diagnosis of haematological conditions are true:

  A a differential white cell count performed by an analyser is accurate provided the cell morphology is normal
  B the neutrophil count tends to be higher in people of African origin than of European origin
  C neutrophilia is more marked in acute viral infections than in bacterial ones
  D the platelet count commonly falls during pregnancy
  E a false low platelet count can be obtained if the blood has been taken into EDTA anticoagulant

10.2 Deficiencies of the following food substances are linked with the following haematological conditions:

  A iron and megaloblastic anaemia
  B cobalamin and haemolytic anaemia
  C folic acid and microcytic anaemia
  D riboflavin and red cell aplasia
  E vitamin C and microcytic, normocytic or macrocytic anaemia

10.3 The following statements about normal iron metabolism are true:

  A the normal daily requirement for adults is 1-2 mg
  B the main site of absorption is the ileum
  C haemoglobin accounts for about 75% of total body iron
  D there is no physiological route for iron excretion
  E iron is more readily absorbed from vegetables than from meat

10.4 Increased red cell destruction has the following pathological effects:

  A raised unconjugated bilirubin
  B raised haptoglobins
  C reduced methaemalbumin
  D increased urinary urobilinogen
  E haemosiderinuria

10. Haematology

10.5 Glucose-6-phosphate dehydrogenase deficiency

A   is a Y-linked trait
B   appears in Afro-caribbean populations as well as Mediterranean, Middle Eastern and Oriental populations
C   may cause acute haemolysis following the ingestion of fava spices
D   can cause neonatal jaundice in affected males
E   is diagnosed definitively by visual microscopic examination of red cells

10.6 Haemolytic disease of the newborn

A   results from the transplacental transfer of maternal antigens which destroy the newborn's cells
B   involving the ABO blood group system is more severe than that of the Rhesus system
C   cannot occur without prior sensitization of the immune system by pregnancy or transfusion
D   can be predicted by measuring the optical density of amniotic fluid
E   should be treated by exchange transfusion if the cord blood bilirubin level is greater than 75 mmol/l

10.7 The following drugs are associated with aplastic anaemia:

A   chloramphenicol
B   penicillamine
C   tetracycline
D   thiazides
E   diclofenac

10.8 The following features indicate a poor prognosis in acute lymphoblastic leukaemia:

A   age under 2 years
B   male sex
C   remission achieved within 4 weeks
D   hepatosplenomegaly
E   CNS involvement

10. Haematology

10.9 The following have a recognized role in the aetiology of acute leukaemia:

A benzene
B Down's syndrome
C human lymphotrophic virus HTLV1
D in vitro fertilization
E Fanconi's anaemia

10.10 The following findings are characteristic of chronic lymphocytic leukaemia:

A the lymphocyte cell morphology is abnormal but the count is normal
B low serum immunoglobulins
C normal bone marrow aspiration and biopsy
D raised serum uric acid
E anaemia

10.11 The following findings are characteristic of chronic granulocytic leukaemia:

A anaemia
B basophilia
C increased platelet count
D raised neutrophil alkaline phosphatase
E low serum vitamin B12

10.12 Chronic lymphocytic leukaemia

A is usually caused by malignant transformation of a T cell
B is the most common leukaemia in the Orient, Europe and the USA
C usually occurs in people aged under 30
D is twice as common in men as women
E during the early stages may not require immediate treatment with chemotherapy

10. Haematology

10.13 The following features are characteristic of myelodysplastic disorders

  A splenomegaly
  B high blood counts
  C basophilia
  D increased marrow cellularity
  E increased marrow dysplasia

10.14 The following conditions are associated with disseminated intravascular coagulation

  A prostatic carcinoma
  B breast carcinoma
  C meningococcal infection
  D miscarriage
  E retained placenta

10.15 Haemophilia A

  A has no effect on levels of Factor VIII in females because they are carriers
  B is not life treatening provided Factor VIII levels remain above 30% of normal activity levels
  C causes a prolonged activated partial thromboplastic time (APTT)
  D can be diagnosed by assaying serum Factor VIII levels
  E may be complicated by chronic joint pain which can be safely treated by ibuprofen

11. IMMUNOLOGY AIDS

11.1 A depressed immune response may result from

  A obesity
  B antibiotic treatment
  C renal failure
  D old age
  E infection

11.2 Disorders associated with HLA-DR3 include

  A ankylosing spondylitis
  B coeliac disease
  C Sjögren's syndrome
  D muscular dystrophy
  E systemic lupus erythematosus (SLE)

11.3 The following clinical problems and infective complications are typically linked together:

  A Hodgkin's disease and *Pseudomonas aeruginosa*
  B AIDS and pneumococcal sepsis
  C burns and varicella zoster
  D aplastic anaemia and Gram-negative rod bacteraemia
  E hyposplenism and *Pneumocystis carinii*

11.4 Important viral infections of immunocompromised patients are caused by

  A candida
  B cytomegalovirus (CMV)
  C varicella zoster
  D aspergillus
  E echoviruses

11. Immunology and AIDS

11.5 The human immunodeficiency virus (HIV)

A is rapidly inactivated by boiling
B can survive for long periods at ambient temperatures on most surfaces
C is rapidly killed by hypochlorite (household bleach)
D can be transmitted by subcutaneous injections using infected instruments
E can be transmitted by Factor VIII despite heat treatment

11.6 Human immunodeficiency virus (HIV) can be transmitted by

A saliva
B needle-stick injury
C breast milk
D sharing cooking facilities
E urine

11.7 The following statements are true of the HIV antibody test:

A the interval between sero-conversion and exposure to infection is usually no more than 2 months
B a seronegative individual can infect other people
C the virus is more readily isolated from blood than other body fluids
D a positive antibody test is always indicative of infection
E detection of antibodies is the cheapest and most accurate of HIV diagnostic procedures

11.8 The following prognostic markers indicate progression of AIDS:

A rising CD4 lymphocytes
B falling ESR
C rising p24 antibody
D falling p24 antigen
E polycythaemia

11. Immunology and AIDS

11.9 The following conditions commonly cause persistent generalized lymphadenopathy:

   A gonorrhoea
   B cytomegalovirus
   C primary syphilis
   D toxoplasmosis
   E sarcoidosis

11.10 In patients with AIDS, Kaposi's sarcoma

   A more commonly affects homosexuals than heterosexuals and haemophiliacs
   B usually presents at a single site initially
   C commonly metastasizes to the brain
   D should be treated early and aggressively to improve prognosis
   E is more aggressive than in the classical or endemic variants

11.11 The following features of *Pneumocystis carinii* pneumonia (PCP) are true:

   A PCP is the presenting feature in 50% of cases of AIDS
   B patients with PCP pursue a rapid downhill course from diagnosis
   C chest radiographs typically show bilateral, diffuse interstitial shadowing
   D a normal chest radiograph is possible in the early stages
   E sputum seldom contains the causative protozoan

11.12 Common haematological abnormalities in patients with AIDS include

   A neutropenia
   B thrombocytosis
   C target cells
   D anaemia
   E raised ESR

11. Immunology and AIDS

11.13 The following statements about AIDS in Africa are true:

    A AIDS is most commonly spread by heterosexual contact
    B African isolates of the virus are more virulent than those from elsewhere
    C the most severe opportunistic infection is tuberculosis
    D *Pneumocystis carinii* pneumonia is less common than in Western countries
    E 'Slim disease' is enteropathic AIDS

11.14 AIDS in children

    A to date, affects less than 100 cases worldwide
    B is usually due to materno-fetal transmission
    C can be excluded in neonates by the enzyme-linked immunosorbent assay (ELISA) test
    D usually presents clinically with nonspecific symptoms
    E excludes immunization with live vaccines

11.15 Zidovudine in the treatment of AIDS

    A has an elimination half-life of 24 hours
    B barely penetrates the blood brain barrier
    C is mainly metabolized in the kidney
    D reduces the incidence and severity of opportunistic infections
    E prolonged gastrointestinal side-effects are common

12. INFECTIONS

12.1 **PUO**

    A when due to infection in developing countries, is most commonly caused by tuberculosis
    B is unlikely to be due to endocarditis if antibiotics have been taken recently
    C may be due to hypernephroma
    D usually needs investigation by laparotomy
    E may be due to drugs

12.2 **Active immunity is induced by**

    A diphtheria vaccine
    B human normal immunoglobulin
    C tetanus toxoid
    D BCG
    E anti-tetanus immunoglobulin

12.3 **Meningococcal meningitis**

    A is the most common type of bacterial meningitis in the UK
    B causes a characteristic rash in most patients
    C is diagnosed by finding Gram-positive cocci in the CSF or blood
    D should be treated by intrathecal benzylpenicillin
    E may cause a septic arthritis

12.4 **Encephalitis can be caused by**

    A herpes simplex
    B arboviruses
    C chickenpox
    D human immunodeficiency virus
    E rabies

12. Infections

12.5 Toxoplasmosis

A occurs commonly in the UK where over half the population has acquired antibody by middle age   T
B is caught by close contact with birds   F
C should be treated in pregnancy with spiramycin   T
D can cause congenital intracranial calcification   T
E can be diagnosed by isolating *T. cruzi* from blood   F

Not cruzi + by IgM IFA Sabin Feldman

12.6 Yersinia entercolitis

A affects both the large and small bowel
B commonly causes a bloody diarrhoea
C can be diagnosed by urine culture
D can cause an acute arthritis
E is generally mild not needing specific treatment

12.7 Typhoid fever

A needs an insect vector   F
B usually causes a neutropenia   T
C is an intracellular infection
D usually affects the gallbladder   T
E is caused by *S. typhi* which multiplies in reticuloendothelial cells   T

lymph Peyers / RE / Blood

12.8 The spores of *Clostridium tetani*

A are quickly destroyed by exposure to fresh air
B contain the active neurotoxin
C can remain within healed wounds to become active later
D germinate to produce a Gram-positive bacillus
E cause infection via minor wounds as commonly as via major wounds

12. Infections

12.9 Brucellosis

- A is a zoonosis
- B can cause a subclinical infection
- C has an incubation period of several days to several months
- D should be treated with penicillin in the first instance
- E can be diagnosed by blood cultures in most patients in the acute phase

12.10 The signs and symptoms of diphtheria include

- A tonsillar lymphadenopathy
- B croup
- C pleurisy
- D chronic skin cancer
- E uveitis

12.11 The following statements are true:

- A *Staphylococcus aureus* is seldom resistant to methicillin
- B ampicillin is the antibiotic of choice for *Haemophilus influenzae* infection
- C most anaerobic bacteria are sensitive to metronidazole
- D aminoglycosides are bacteriostatic
- E in the presence of inflammation chloramphenicol penetrates the meninges poorly

12.12 Aminoglycosides

- A are effective by interrupting bacterial protein synthesis
- B are inactivated by gastric acid
- C include streptomycin
- D should be tailored according to liver function tests
- E may be ototoxic

12. Infections

12.13 The following antibiotics and side-effects are linked together:

A penicillin and Stevens-Johnson syndrome
B aminoglycosides and tooth pigmentation
C sulphonamides and Stevens-Johnson syndrome
D chloramphenicol and aplastic anaemia
E metronidazole and pseudomembranous colitis

12.14 Herpes encephalitis

A nearly always affects the temporal lobes
B causes focal fits early in the disease
C if untreated has a 75% mortality
D may require brain biopsy for definitive diagnosis
E can run a mild course and never be diagnosed

12.15 The Epstein-Barr virus

A is found in at least 50% of children in developed countries
B is a togavirus
C has been closely linked with the pathogenesis of leukaemias
D causes infectious mononucleosis
E can be caught by sharing eating utensils

12.16 Measles

A accounts for 15 per cent of deaths from all causes in children under five in developed countries
B may cause recurrent pneumothoraces
C may cause corneal ulceration
D is more dangerous in overcrowded households
E establishes lifelong immunity after natural infection

51

12. Infections

12.17 Recognized features of Lyme disease include

- A erythema nodosum
- B arthritis
- C pancarditis
- D polyneuritis
- E pleurisy

12.18 The following statements are true of polio vaccination:

- A Salk inactivated polio vaccine produces humoral immunity but no detectable secretory IgA antibodies
- B Sabin oral live attenuated vaccine stimulates both serum antibodies and local secretory IgA antibodies
- C immunization should be delayed in a child with any minor infectious disease
- D pregnancy is an absolute contraindication to immunization
- E immunosuppressed individuals should receive the live, oral vaccine rather than the injected, inactivated vaccine

12.19 Recognised complications of rabies include

- A pneumothorax
- B diabetes mellitus
- C cardiac arrhythmias
- D sensory neuropathy
- E cerebral oedema

12.20 The following statements about anthrax are true:

- A untreated, cutaneous anthrax is fatal in up to 20% of patients
- B anthrax spores will not survive cooking
- C *Bacillus anthracis* can seldom be isolated from the sputum of patients with pulmonary anthrax
- D benzylpenicillin is the treatment of choice for all types of anthrax
- E gastrointestinal anthrax is a mild form with a low mortality

12. Infections

12.21 The following are useful in protection against malaria:

    A mosquito nets T
    B chloroquine T
    C tonic water F
    D pyridoxine F
    E tretinoin F

12.22 Dengue fever *yellow flavoured dengue viral*

    A is transmitted by droplet infection F
    B is associated typically with a lymphocytosis F
    C is self-limiting and almost never fatal F
    D is associated with lymphadenopathy and splenomegaly
    E shows a diagnostic increase in dengue virus haemagglutination inhibition antibody T

12.23 The following are effective treatments for typhus:

    A cotrimoxazole
    B metronidazole
    C pentamidine
    D chloramphenicol
    E tetracycline

12.24 The following statements are true of hydatid disease:

    A the two species commonly infecting man are *Echinococcus grandiosa* and *Echinococcus unilocularis*
    B humans become infected by eating contaminated pork
    C the tapeworm embryo reaches its final destination via the portal circulation
    D more than 75% of hydatid cysts occur in the liver
    E the Casoni test is a reliable diagnostic test

12. Infections

12.25 The symptoms and signs of lymphatic filariasis include

   A epididymitis
   B hydrocele
   C chyluria
   D asthma
   E heart failure

12.26 The following investigations are useful in the diagnosis of loiasis:

   A white blood cell count
   B daytime 'fresh' thick blood film
   C pleural biopsy
   D the Mantoux test
   E fixation of a blood film and staining with Mayer's haemalum

12.27 Onchocerciasis

   A is transmitted by the tsetse fly
   B has an important animal reservoir in the baboon
   C is most prevalent in persons living near fast-flowing streams
   D may present with subcutaneous nodules over bony points
   E could be eradicated by a worldwide programme of chemoprophylaxis

12.28 Intestinal schistosomiasis

   A is mainly caused by *S. haematobium*
   B is common in coastal areas where sea water harbours the specific, snail host
   C often causes an eosinophilia
   D is effectively treated by praziquantel or oxamniquine
   E may cause no symptoms in previously exposed individuals

12. Infections

12.29 Leptospirosis

    A is caused by *L. interrogans*, a highly motile spirochaete
    B has an incubation period of about three months
    C can cause interstitial nephritis
    D usually causes jaundice
    E in pregnancy has a high fetal mortality

12.30 The clinical features of leprosy include

    A endomyocardial fibrosis
    B foot drop
    C lagophthalmos
    D hypopigmented macules
    E testicular atrophy

12.31 In the treatment of plague

    A penicillin is the most effective drug
    B streptomycin is contraindicated if the patient develops renal failure
    C chloramphenicol is indicated for patients with meningitis
    D antibiotic resistance is common, necessitating multiple drug regimes
    E buboes seldom recede without incision and drainage

13. LIVER DISEASE

13.1 The following statements about liver metabolism are true:

  A urinary urobilinogen is a nonspecific test of obstructive jaundice
  B two thirds of circulating bilirubin is metabolized by the liver, the remainder by the kidney
  C bilirubin is transported in the circulation bound to globulin
  D conjugated bilirubin is water soluble
  E most urobilinogen is excreted in the faeces

13.2 The following statements about the investigation of the liver and biliary tract are true:

  A oral cholecystography is a useful investigation of a jaundiced patient
  B nuclear medicine studies are the best investigation of liver parenchyma
  C most gallstones are radio-opaque
  D endoscopic retrograde cholangio-pancreatography is the best method of demonstrating stones in the common bile duct
  E liver secondary tumours are usually highly vascular and well visualized by angiography

13.3 Hepatitis E

  A is transmitted by contaminated needles and blood transfusions
  B often progresses to chronic hepatitis
  C is linked with disseminated intravascular coagulation in pregnant women
  D is the new name for non-A, non-B hepatitis
  E has a mortality of less than 5%

13.4 The following liver diseases are caused by protozoa:

  A amoebiasis
  B hydatid disease
  C Wilson's disease
  D leishmaniasis
  E malaria

13. Liver Disease

13.5 **Hepatic amoebiasis**

　A　is transmitted to humans via the dog which is the intermediate host
　B　should be routinely investigated by needle aspiration of a suspected abscess
　C　is caused by the protozoa *Echinococcus histolytica*
　D　should be treated by metronidazole or tinidazole in the first instance
　E　is commonly found in temperate zones

13.6 **The following features are characteristic of unconjugated hyperbilirubinaemia in infancy:**

　A　hepatomegaly
　B　pale stools
　C　normal liver function tests
　D　bilirubin in the urine
　E　jaundice

13.7 **The causes of prehepatic jaundice in childhood include**

　A　Gilbert's syndrome
　B　Epstein-Barr virus infection
　C　exposure to halothane
　D　haemolysis
　E　Wilson's disease

13.8 **The causes of chronic hepatitis include**

　A　hepatitis C
　B　Wilson's disease
　C　propranolol
　D　methyldopa
　E　systemic lupus erythematosus

13. Liver Disease

13.9 Primary biliary cirrhosis

    A affects women more than men
    B is found more commonly in tropical rather than in temperate climates
    C can be reliably diagnosed by testing for antinuclear factor
    D should be treated with long-term corticosteroids
    E is linked with osteoporosis

13.10 The following are vasoactive drugs useful in the treatment of bleeding oesophageal varices:

    A vasopressin
    B somatostatin
    C nitroglycerin
    D angiotensin
    E glypressin

13.11 Hepatic ascites results from a combination of

    A decreased plasma colloid pressure
    B systemic hypertension
    C increased hepatic lymph production
    D reduced hepatic venous flow
    E reduced albumin synthesis in the liver

13.12 The following statements about gallstones are true:

    A cholesterol stones are strongly associated with bacteria in the bile
    B the incidence of stones in the gallbladder rises with age
    C few stones remain symptomless
    D treatment with chenodeoxycholic acid may be effective for pigment stones
    E cholecystectomy is the standard treatment for symptomatic gallstones

13. Liver Disease

13.13 Hepatocellular carcinoma

    A is linked to cirrhosis
    B is linked to schistosomiasis
    C is one of the most common malignancies in the Orient and sub-Saharan Africa
    D is characterized by high levels of α-fetoprotein
    E is best diagnosed by liver biopsy

13.14 The causes of Budd-Chiari syndrome include

    A polycythaemia rubra vera
    B hypernephroma
    C hormone replacement therapy
    D alcoholic hepatitis
    E cirrhosis

13.15 The causes of portal hypertension include

    A mesenteric venous thrombosis
    B portal venous thrombosis
    C splenic venous thrombosis
    D secondary liver metastases
    E ascites

14. MULTISYSTEM DISORDERS

14.1 **The following statements about systemic lupus erythematosus are true:**

　A　women are affected more commonly than men
　B　concordance between identical twins is low
　C　the combined oral contraceptive pill often improves symptoms
　D　antinuclear antibody (ANA) is a useful diagnostic test
　E　chloroquine has been superseded by cyclophosphamide in the treatment of mild disease

14.2 **Scleroderma may present with**

　A　Raynaud's phenomenon
　B　pulmonary hypertension
　C　proteinuria
　D　peripheral neuropathy
　E　telangiectasia

14.3 **The features of systemic amyloidosis include**

　A　proteinuria
　B　heart block
　C　macroglossia
　D　purpura
　E　peripheral neuropathy

14.4 **Polyarteritis nodosa**

　A　primarily affects large arteries
　B　is more common in males than in females
　C　seldom affects veins
　D　presents more commonly in people over 60 years of age than in younger age groups
　E　is no longer treated with prednisolone because the dangers outweigh the benefits

15. NEUROLOGY

15.1 The following statements about migraine are true:

    A over half of all patients have their first attack before the age of 20
    B over half of all patients have an aura before the headache
    C frequency of attacks may vary from occasional to daily
    D to make the diagnosis of migraine the headache must be unilateral
    E vasoconstriction of cerebral blood vessels is characteristic of migraine

15.2 The EEG

    A is poor at precisely localizing a cerebral lesion
    B is required for the diagnosis for brain stem death in the UK
    C suffers from high variability in infants, making interpretation difficult
    D is rarely helpful in the diagnosis of dementia
    E is normal between epileptic attacks in most epileptic patients

15.3 The following facts about the EEG are true:

    A a normal EEG effectively excludes epilepsy
    B sharp wave paroxysmal activity is associated with epilepsy
    C a normal EEG excludes acute encephalitis
    D structural abnormalities not detected by CT scanning or magnetic resonance imaging can be detected by EEG
    E the EEG is usually normal in patients with cerebral dysfunction caused by drugs

15.4 The following muscle groups are supplied by the following peripheral nerves:

    A biceps by the musculocutaneous nerve
    B interossei by the median nerve
    C quadriceps by the sciatic nerve
    D gastrocnemius by the femoral nerve
    E triceps by the radial nerve

15. Neurology

15.5 Lumbar puncture

A in acutely ill patients should generally be preceded by a CT scan
B is performed by passing a needle into the subarachnoid space at the level of the termination of the spinal cord
C has risks, of which passing the needle too far into the aorta is a common one
D is safe in patients with suspected intracranial masses provided there is no papilloedema
E is safe in patients with raised intracranial pressure due to a communication hydrocephalus

15.6 Multiple sclerosis

A has a higher prevalence in tropical zones than in temperate zones
B presents as a single symptom in most patients
C may present with diplopia due to optic nerve involvement
D does not cause progressive disability in up to one third of patients
E very rarely causes sensory disturbance of the limbs

15.7 The spasticity of multiple sclerosis can be treated by

A carbamazepine
B oxybutynin
C baclofen
D dantrolene sodium
E calcium antagonists

15.8 The following conditions are among those necessary for a diagnosis of brain death to be made in the UK:

A decerebrate posturing (extension of limbs)
B decorticate posturing (flexion of arms, extension of legs)
C fixed pupils
D loss of light reflex
E absent jaw jerk

15. Neurology

15.9 The following conditions are accepted causes of epileptic fits:

    A hypercalcaemia
    B hypernatraemia
    C hyperglycaemia
    D encephalitis
    E systemic lupus erythematosus

15.10 The following side-effects are linked to the following drugs:

    A diplopia and carbamazepine
    B hirsutisim and phenobarbitone
    C hyperammonaemia and sodium valproate
    D phenytoin and weight gain
    E metabolic bone disease and ethosuximide

15.11 Intracranial aneurysms

    A are linked to the presence of hypertension in a significant proportion of patients
    B are seldom familial
    C form most commonly on the anterior communicating artery
    D are multiple in over 50 per cent of patients
    E occur most commonly in the age group 40-60

15.12 Arteriovenous malformations

    A usually cause intracerebral rather than subarachnoid bleeding
    B have a worse prognosis than intracerebral aneurysms
    C almost never affect the cerebellum
    D may present as epilepsy
    E require urgent prophylactic surgery in most cases

15.13 Meningiomas

    A are benign tumours
    B are the most common primary intracranial tumour
    C occur more commonly in those aged under 40 than those over 40
    D respond to radiotherapy
    E almost never recur following surgical resection

15.14 Stroke

- A is the third most common cause of death in the UK
- B is more commonly caused by infarction than haemorrhage
- C is more common among people from socio-economic classes A and B than C and D
- D is more likely to be fatal if caused by infarction than haemorrhage
- E is linked to raised systolic blood pressure but not diastolic

15.15 The following areas are supplied by the following arteries:

- A the parietal lobe is supplied by the posterior inferior cerebellar artery
- B the anterior medial frontal lobe is supplied by the posterior cerebral artery
- C the occipital lobe is supplied by the posterior cerebral artery
- D the retina is supplied by the optic artery
- E the inferior cerebellum is supplied by the middle cerebral artery

15.16 The side-effects of pyridostigmine include

- A pupillary dilatation
- B constipation
- C dry mouth
- D colic
- E increased sweating

15.17 Duchenne muscular dystrophy

- A is the most common primary muscle cell disease in the developed world
- B is very rarely the result of a new mutation
- C is an X-linked disorder
- D usually causes death in affected patients before the age of 20
- E is characterized by the presence of dystrophin in the muscle fibres

15. Neurology

15.18 The tremor of idiopathic Parkinsonism

- A is rarely the presenting feature
- B tends to affect proximal muscle groups rather than distal ones
- C is very rarely unilateral
- D may temporarily by improved by movement
- E may produce flexion-extension movements of the fingers

15.19 The recognized features of idiopathic Parkinsonism include

- A hyperkinesia
- B hypersecretion
- C dysphagia
- D lack of blinking
- E impaired ocular convergence

15.20 The following statements about motor neurone disease are true:

- A the cause in unknown
- B middle aged people between 40 and 60 are more commonly affected than younger or older people
- C most patients survive less than 5 years following diagnosis
- D treatment progression is unaltered by treatment
- E most patients die from gastrointestinal complications

15.21 The following conditions may cause acute facial palsy:

- A sarcoidosis
- B Guillain-Barre syndrome
- C Lyme disease
- D motor neurone disease
- E HIV infection

15. Neurology

15.22 The recognized causes of simultaneous bilateral facial weakness include

A idiopathic Bell's palsy
B sarcoidosis
C Lyme disease
D HIV infection
E subacute sclerosing erythematosus

15.23 The following symptoms are commonly associated with Bell's palsy:

A dry eye
B hyperacusis
C dry mouth
D loss of taste
E postauricular pain

16. NUTRITION

16.1 **The following statements about nutrition are true:**

  A starchy foods are almost as fattening as fatty foods
  B vegetarians live longer than carnivores
  C being overweight is a familial condition
  D individuals who are overweight have a lower basal metabolic rate than people who are normal weight
  E children need to eat sugar for energy levels to be adequate

16.2 **The following statements about breast-feeding are true:**

  A foremilk contains more fat than hindmilk
  B human milk is low in protein compared with cows' milk
  C cows' milk and human milk have similar fat contents
  D vitamin K levels are low in breast milk
  E an exclusively breast-fed infant's iron stores become low 1 month postnatally

16.3 **The following are contraindications to breast feeding:**

  A maternal medication with ampicillin
  B maternal alcoholism
  C phenylketonuria
  D maternal AIDS
  E galactosaemia in the infant

16.4 **The clinical features of marasmus include**

  A severe wasting
  B no oedema
  C severe muscle wasting
  D dystrophic changes of nails
  E normal growth in children

67

16.5 The clinical features of kwashiorkor include

    A splenomegaly
    B oedema
    C subcutaneous fat present
    D constipation
    E muscle wasting

16.6 Congestive cardiac failure has been linked with deficiency of

    A selenium
    B zinc
    C thiamine
    D vitamin D
    E riboflavin

16.7 The following types of food additives are permitted in the UK:

    A preservatives with E numbers
    B saccharin
    C emulsifiers
    D cobalt salts
    E antioxidants

17. ONCOLOGY

17.1 The following drugs can cause necrosis if they infiltrate local tissues:

   A   doxorubicin
   B   cyclosporin
   C   mustine
   D   vincristine
   E   dexamethasone

17.2 Radiotherapy is the treatment of choice for the following tumours:

   A   early squamous cell carcinoma of the skin
   B   locally advanced cervical carcinoma
   C   Hodgkin's disease
   D   vaginal carcinoma
   E   early anal carcinoma

17.3 The characteristic clinical features of malignant hypercalcaemia include

   A   diarrhoea
   B   peripheral sensory neuropathy
   C   renal failure caused by anuria
   D   muscle weakness
   E   tetany

17.4 Malignant hypercalcaemia

   A   is the most common life-threatening metabolic disorder associated with cancer
   B   is usually due to carcinoma of the bowel
   C   may occur in the absence of overt bone disease
   D   should be treated in the first instance by mithramycin
   E   is caused by the ectopic secretion of parathyroid hormone for reasons not understood

17. Oncology

17.5 Cerebral metastases

A are the most common space-occupying lesion of the brain
B are solitary, at the time of diagnosis, in about 50% of cases
C affect the cerebellum more commonly than the hemispheres
D occur early in the natural history of melanoma
E typically occur at the junction of the grey and white matter

17.6 The following signs may occur in superior vena caval obstruction:

A distension of superficial thoracic veins
B swelling of the tongue
C nerve deafness
D proptosis
E conjunctival oedema

17.7 Neutropenia is typically found in the following cancers:

A brain
B breast
C prostate
D lymphoma
E lung

17.8 Breast cancer

A is the most common malignant tumour of Western women
B is becoming increasingly rare in developing countries
C should be diagnosed by open biopsy in most cases
D in women with advanced disease is most successfully treated with chemotherapy alone
E causes up to 35% of women to suffer from severe anxiety and depression if they need surgery

17. Oncology

17.9 The following factors have been positively linked with breast cancer:

A onset of menstruation after 15 years of age
B obesity
C high alcohol consumption
D low socio-economic status in developed countries
E age over 30 years at birth of first child, provided there have been no previous incomplete pregnancies

17.10 The following factors are positively associated with cancer of the cervix:

A cervical intra-epithelial neoplasia
B teenage sexual intercourse
C barrier methods of contraception
D increasing parity
E smoking

17.11 The following statements about cervical cancer are true:

A most cervical cancers are squamous in type
B blood borne metastases are more common than lymph spread
C almost one half of all patients with cancer of the cervix suffer a local recurrence
D whenever a nation introduces screening there has been a fall in both mortality and morbidity
E small (less than 50 mm diameter) volume disease has as much metastatic potential as larger disease

17.12 Endometrial cancer

A is more common among women using progestogen containing oral contraceptives
B is usually poorly differentiated
C is now most effectively treated by a combination of radiotherapy and hormone based chemotherapy
D is characterized by late blood borne metastasis, usually to the lung
E has usually spread to local lymph glands at diagnosis

17. Oncology

17.13 Ovarian cancer

- A occurs more commonly among women with breast cancer than in the general population
- B occurs in some families as an autosomal dominant trait
- C is less common among Japanese women than North Americans
- D occurs in parous women more commonly than in nulliparous women
- E is more common among women who used hormone replacement therapy without a progestogen component

17.14 The following statements about bladder cancer are correct:

- A bladder cancer is usually a papilliferous squamous carcinoma
- B at presentation, most tumours have invaded the muscle of the bladder wall
- C survival correlates well with TNM staging at presentation
- D superficial tumours, if effectively treated by endoscopic resection and diathermy, seldom become invasive
- E chemotherapy for metastatic disease is ineffective and seldom used

17.15 Prostatic cancer

- A is seldom seen in men under the age of 50
- B is usually a poorly differentiated cancer
- C can be accurately diagnosed using prostate-specific antigen
- D can be treated by radiotherapy in the early stages as effectively as by surgery
- E responds objectively in almost all cases to hormone therapy

17.16 Multiple myeloma has the following effects:

- A it suppresses antibody formation
- B it activates osteoblasts to destroy bone
- C it stimulates marrow function
- D it can cause amyloid formation
- E it stimulates the production of Bence-Jones protein in the blood

17. Oncology

17.17 Multiple myeloma

- A is a malignancy of the T lymphocyte lineage
- B is more common in white populations than black
- C occurs as commonly in those under 65 as in those over 65
- D commonly presents as bone fractures which are pain free
- E is linked with plasma cell leukaemia

17.18 The following statements about Hodgkin's disease are true:

- A the Reed-Sternberg cell is no longer regarded as the significant malignant cell
- B the nodular sclerotic subtype is the most common histological type
- C the disease is best diagnosed by bone marrow biopsy
- D a staging laparotomy is indicated in most patients
- E survival has been improved in patients with early disease following the addition of chemotherapy to radiotherapy

17.19 The following statements about bone tumours are true:

- A the most common bone tumour is chondrosarcoma
- B most tumours affect the ends of long bones
- C radiology will fail to detect as many as 30% of bone tumours
- D bone tumours seldom metastasize to lymph nodes
- E surgery, in combination with radiotherapy, is the treatment of choice for most tumours

17.20 The following single gene disorders are associated with an increased incidence of paediatric neoplasia:

- A tuberose sclerosis
- B adrenogenital syndrome
- C Fanconi's anaemia
- D ataxia telangiectasia
- E Pick's disease

17. Oncology

17.21 The following functions can be adversely affected by treatment for childhood malignancy:
- A hearing by cisplatin
- B cardiac function by aminoglycosides
- C pulmonary function by anthracyclines
- D renal function by methotrexate
- E thyroid function by radiation

18. ORAL MEDICINE

18.1 The following drugs are associated with gingival swelling:

  A methyldopa
  B cyclosporin
  C phenytoin
  D amantadine
  E nifedipine

18.2 The causes of pigmented mucosal lesions of the mouth include

  A Plummer-Vinson syndrome
  B systemic lupus erythematosus
  C benzodiazepines
  D Kaposi's sarcoma
  E haemochromatosis

18.3 The following predispose to oral cancer:

  A high alcohol consumption
  B smoking cigarettes
  C folate deficiency
  D tea drinking
  E cigar smoking

18.4 The following drugs cause a dry mouth:

  A monoamine oxidase inhibitors
  B antihistamines
  C bronchoconstrictors
  D phenothiazines
  E amphetamines

19. POISONING

19.1 The following statements about acute poisoning are true:

    A intentional self-poisoning is the second most common cause of death in the first four decades of life
    B the lowest incidence of poisoning occurs in the pre-adolescent (6-12 years) group
    C girls are more likely to succeed in committing suicide than boys
    D about 10 per cent of adolescents repeat self-poisoning
    E the incidence of intentional self-poisoning is lower in the over 60 age group than for the general population

19.2 Overdoses of the following substances can be treated with the antidote listed:

    A β-blockers by glucagon
    B warfarin by protamine
    C benzodiazepines by penicillamine
    D opioids by naloxone
    E lead by flumazenil

19.3 Activated charcoal

    A is the best absorbent currently available
    B is valuable in the treatment of poisoning by acids and alkalis
    C is not effective if administered more than 1 hour following ingestion of a poison
    D is more effective than syrup of ipecacuanha in preventing poison absorption
    E is valuable in the treatment of ethanol overdosage

19.4 Features of salicylate overdose include

    A hypertension
    B bradycardia
    C hyperventilation
    D deafness
    E sweating

19. Poisoning

19.5 The following statements about some of the clinical sequelae of theophylline poisoning are true:

A nausea and vomiting are due to stimulation of the medullary vomiting centre
B hypotension is due to decreased cardiac output
C hyperventilation is due to inhibition of medullary respiratory centres
D respiratory alkalosis is due to hyperventilation
E diarrhoea is due to a local gastrointestinal effect

19.6 The following statements about poisoning are true:

A a chest radiograph is indicated in every person who has swallowed a disc (button) battery
B liquid detergents cause few toxic effects other than nausea, vomiting and diarrhoea
C the most toxic effects of petroleum distillates are respiratory
D ingestion of strong acids should be treated by gastric emptying and lavage
E erythrocyte cholinesterase activity is a good measure of the severity of acute organophosphate poisoning

19.7 The recognized characteristic features of acute lithium poisoning include

A constipation
B hyperkalaemia
C hypertension
D nystagmus
E cardiac rhythm disturbances

20. PSYCHIATRY

20.1 The following factors predispose to major depression:

    A social groups A and B
    B a first degree relative with major depression
    C the presence of more than 3 children in the home
    D employment in the same company for more than 10 years
    E loss of a parent before 11 years of age

20.2 ECT in the treatment of depression

    A is indicated if vegetative symptoms, such as early morning waking, are present
    B is contraindicated in the presence of psychotic symptoms
    C is a safe procedure with a mortality of less than 0.1% for each course of treatment
    D causes short-term memory loss which is usually permanent
    E must cause a seizure to be effective

20.3 The following are good prognostic indicators in schizophrenia:

    A known precipitating cause
    B no affective symptoms
    C no catatonic symptoms
    D gradual onset
    E prompt treatment

20.4 The following statements about schizophrenia are true:

    A the incidence of lifetime first schizophrenic illness is broadly similar worldwide across different cultures
    B the peak incidence of schizophrenia is 25-30 years of age
    C in Western countries schizophrenia is most common among lower socio-economic groups
    D in the UK more than 50% of patients are still in hospital two years following admission
    E recent research has shown that schizophrenia is an autosomal dominant illness

20. Psychiatry

20.5 Drugs within the following groups commonly react unfavourably with lithium:

A ACE inhibitors
B 5-HT antagonists
C morphine-based substances
D diuretics
E non-steroidal anti-inflammatory drugs

20.6 The recognized side-effects of 5-HT uptake inhibitors include

A drowsiness
B increased appetite
C anxiety
D sweating
E seizures

20.7 The adverse effects of lithium include

A coarse tremor
B hypoglycaemia
C polyuria
D neutropenia
E hypothyroidism

20.8 The adverse side-effects of tricyclic antidepressants include

A blurred vision
B hyperactivity
C weight gain
D bradycardia
E constipation

20.9 Postnatal depression

A occurs in up to 25% of women after giving birth
B is more common in women with a history of psychiatric illness
C is more common in women who have had obstetric complications
D results in suicide attempts by up to 10% of affected women
E in breast feeding mothers cannot be treated by antidepressant drugs because they are secreted into breast milk in large amounts

20.10 Puerperal psychosis

A is affective in nature
B begins about three months post-partum
C may be complicated by hallucinations
D usually has to be managed by separating the mother from her baby because of the danger she poses to her baby
E on average takes a year before recovery is evident

20.11 The characteristics of the family that may predispose it to violence to children include

A the husband is violent to the wife so the wife is violent to the children
B the children are taught that it is acceptable to hit people who are loved
C the family has not been stressed by major life events
D the family spends much more time interacting with each other than with others
E the intensity of family emotional involvement is very high

20.12 Inhaling solvents

A usually causes a withdrawn, somnolent state in the short term
B causes effects which last 12-24 hours
C causes a characteristic smell on the breath
D may cause renal failure in the regular user
E is possible from a crisp packet

20. Psychiatry

20.13 The following statements about bulimia nervosa are true:

- A bulimia nervosa is less common among women than anorexia nervosa
- B patients usually present looking markedly underweight and emaciated
- C patients rarely have problems with other forms of abuse such as alcohol or drugs
- D many patients display parotid gland enlargement
- E some patients will respond favourably to antidepressive medication

20.14 People with Down's syndrome are particularly prone to

- A diabetes insipidus
- B hypothyroidism
- C hyperparathyroidism
- D Alzheimer's disease
- E Addison's disease

21. RENAL DISORDERS

21.1 The following factors may raise the plasma creatinine level:

    A   any disease which reduces muscle mass
    B   ketones
    C   cephalosporins
    D   aspirin
    E   co-trimoxazole

21.2 The plasma urea is raised by

    A   tetracycline
    B   hepatitis
    C   severe infections
    D   doxycycline
    E   high glucocorticoid dosage

21.3 Patients with the following diseases should not be deprived of fluids before an intravenous urogram:

    A   myelomatosis
    B   scleroderma
    C   diabetes
    D   polycythaemia rubra vera
    E   nephrotic syndrome

21.4 Renal ultrasound

    A   is a sensitive method of detecting hydronephrosis
    B   does not delineate renal parenchyma well
    C   is particularly useful for detecting small lesions in the pelvicalyceal system
    D   cannot usually detect perirenal collections because of overlying gas-filled bowel
    E   cannot detect non-opaque stones

21. Renal Disorders

21.5 In the following situations percutaneous renal biopsy is contraindicated or unnecessary:

A nephrotic syndrome
B cystic kidney disease
C nephrolithiasis
D proteinuria
E end-stage renal failure

21.6 The following statements about renal biopsy are true:

A the lateral border of the lower pole is the safest part to biopsy
B bleeding is the most common complication
C the presence of the nephrotic syndrome is a contraindication to biopsy
D a small, shrunken kidney is easy to biopsy because it does not move much with respiration
E intravenous diazepam during the procedure is contraindicated

21.7 During normal pregnancy

A the effective renal plasma flow falls
B the glomerular filtration rate rises
C the diastolic blood pressure falls by about 15 mm Hg
D bacteriuria has an excellent prognosis and therefore does not usually require antimicrobial treatment
E there is an increased risk of renal calculi

21.8 Pre-eclampsia

A usually occurs after the 20th week of pregnancy
B is more common in second pregnancies than in first
C is the most common cause of hypertension in pregnancy
D is characterized by proteinuria and oedema
E can be successfully treated by methyldopa

21. Renal Disorders

21.9 The following organisms can cause glomerulonephritis:

   A *Mycobacterium leprae*
   B *Wucheria bancrofti*
   C *Actinomyces israeli*
   D *Plasmodium malariae*
   E *Loa-loa*

21.10 The consequences of glomerular dysfunction include

   A postural hypotension
   B hypocoagulability
   C hypercalcaemia
   D low density hyperlipoproteinaemia
   E hypocholesterolaemia

21.11 The following side-effects are linked with the specified drug:

   A muscle cramps and atenolol
   B fluid retention and verapamil
   C cutaneous flushing and frusemide
   D impotence and propranolol
   E hirsutism and captopril

21.12 The side-effects of cyclosporin include

   A cataracts
   B hyperglycaemia
   C hirsutism
   D gingival hyperplasia
   E nephrotoxicity

21. Renal Disorders

21.13 The advantages of continuous ambulatory peritoneal dialysis include

- A absence of haemodynamic fluctuations during dialysis
- B absence of infective complications
- C improvement in pre-existing hyperlipidaemia in some patients
- D improved growth rates in children compared with haemodialysis
- E less rigorous fluid and dietary restrictions compared with haemodialysis

21.14 The following drugs can cause acute tubular necrosis:

- A sulphonamides
- B tetracyclines
- C cephalosporins
- D aminoglycosides
- E co-trimoxazole

21.15 The following statements about nocturnal enuresis are true:

- A most children with nocturnal enuresis are reliably dry during the day
- B by the age of 10 years only about 1% of children suffer nocturnal enuresis
- C first born children are more prone to nocturnal enuresis than later children
- D urodynamic studies can often help diagnose the cause of nocturnal enuresis
- E tricyclic drugs are effective by reason of their anticholinergic and antidepressant effects

21.16 The following disorders have the specified inheritance:

- A cystinosis in an X-linked disorder
- B Hartnup's disease is an autosomal dominant disorder
- C Meckel's syndrome is an autosomal recessive disorder
- D renal tubular acidosis can be an autosomal dominant or a recessive disorder
- E familial hypophosphataemia is a Y-linked disorder

21. Renal Disorders

21.17 Fanconi's syndrome is characterized by

    A aminoaciduria
    B excess urinary potassium
    C glycosuria
    D renal tubular alkalosis
    E phosphaturia

21.18 Urinary tract infection

    A affects approximately 75% of all women at some stage in their lives
    B has become less common following the introduction of antimicrobial agents
    C is more common in women over 65 years than in men over 65 years
    D is usually caused by multiple organism infections
    E following catheterization is often caused by *Proteus* spp.

21.19 Childhood urinary tract infection

    A has a benign outcome in most children
    B is diagnosed once culture of fresh urine yields pure bacterial growth of greater than 10^3/ml
    C is associated with vesicoureteric reflux in 2 out of 3 affected children
    D is caused by an unsuspected surgical disorder in 5% of children
    E should be treated by combination antimicrobial therapy

21.20 Patients with the following disorders are prone to urate stones:

    A renal tubular acidosis
    B psoriasis
    C leukaemia
    D meduallary sponge kidney
    E ileostomy

21. Renal Disorders

21.21 **The following statements about urinary catheterization are correct:**

A silicone coated latex catheters are best suited for long term drainage
B a 12F catheter has an external diameter of 12 millimetres
C the curved-tip Tiemann catheter is effective for men with prostatic obstruction
D the whistle-tip catheter is used for bladder syringing for clot retention
E a 5 ml balloon is adequate to retain the catheter safely in most men

21.22 **Renal cell carcinoma**

A is the most common renal tumour in children
B arises from cells of the distal convoluted tubule
C may present with fever
D may present with hypocalcaemia due to parathyroid hormone production
E may present with erythrocytosis

22. RESPIRATORY DISORDERS

22.1 The following statements about respiratory diseases are true:

A the genetic mutation responsible for most cases of North European cystic fibrosis has been identified
B the likelihood of developing lung cancer is unrelated to genctic factors
C there is a strong association between parental smoking and respiratory infections in their adolescent children
D in the UK about 1 in 10 male deaths is due to lung cancer
E about one third of worldwide deaths from lung cancer occur in developing countries

22.2 The causes of septal lines on chest radiograms include

A lymphangitis carcinomatosis
B allergic aspergillosis
C pneumoconiosis
D hydatid disease
E pulmonary haemosiderosis

22.3 The causes of pleural effusion include

A pancreatitis
B asbestosis
C nephrotic syndrome
D nitrofurantoin
E nephrotic syndrome

22.4 The following statements are true:

A halving the radius of an airway causes a 16-fold reduction in flow
B in health, the small pulmonary airways make the main contribution to airways resistance
C reducing the density of a gas reduces its flow along a tube
D conditions which increase pulmonary compliance generally increase airflow
E the lung volume in an average man is about 6 litres

22. Respiratory Disorders

22.5 Carbon monoxide gas transfer (TLCO) is reduced in the presence of

    A polycythaemia
    B alveolar haemorrhage
    C pneumonia
    D emphysema
    E pulmonary fibrosis

22.6 Contraindications to elective bronchoalveolar lavage include

    A proved myocardial infarction at any time
    B chest infection within the last 6 weeks
    C asthma
    D an FEV1 less than 1.0 litre
    E β-blocker therapy

22.7 The following statements about fibreoptic bronchoscopy are true:

    A the nose provides easier access to the larynx than the mouth
    B with the standard 5mm diameter bronchoscope it is possible to inspect all lobes to sub-segmental level
    C peripheral lesions can be biopsied using paediatric 3.5 mm bronchoscopes
    D no more than one third of lung cancers are visible at bronchoscopy
    E fibreoptic bronchoscopy has a complication rate of less than 1%

22.8 The following are recognized complications of the specified drugs:

    A acute pulmonary oedema and hydralazine
    B reactive eosinophilia and sulphonamides
    C alveolitis and hydrochlorothiazide
    D lupus syndrome and azathioprine
    E oculomucocutaneous syndrome and practolol

22. Respiratory Disorders

22.9 **Acute stridor and epiglottitis**

A is usually caused by a streptococcal infection
B most commonly affects children aged 5-7 years
C should usually be managed in hospital
D is best diagnosed by clinical examination of the throat and a lateral radiograph of the neck
E often recurs

22.10 **The following statements about the investigation of suspected foreign body inhalation are true:**

A initial chest radiograph may be normal, but may be abnormal when repeated later
B in over 50% of cases the chest radiograph provides some diagnostic clues
C in 10% of cases the foreign body is radio-opaque
D radiographs in expiration should be used in preference to radiographs in inspiration
E CT scanning is helpful for the investigation of peripheral lung parenchyma

22.11 **In cystic fibrosis**

A pulmonary disease is present at birth
B pulmonary disease is most commonly found in the right upper lobe
C the primary pulmonary physiological abnormality is large airway obstruction
D the pulmonary vital capacity falls
E the pulmonary residual volume falls

22. Respiratory Disorders

22.12 The following facts about the investigation of asthma in children are true:

- A skin allergy tests are often diagnostic of the precipitating cause
- B chest radiographs are indicated whenever there is an acute episode
- C pulmonary function tests are useful in children over 2 years of age
- D FEV_1 is more reliable in demonstrating airways obstruction than peak expiratory flow
- E IgE and radio-allergosorbent tests are indicated, if available

22.13 In occupational asthma, there is a link between the following occupations and precipitating agents:

- A baking and rye
- B car spray-painting and nickel
- C metal plating and isocyanates
- D nursing and psyllium
- E working in the electronics industry and colophony

22.14 The following are risk factors for the development of chronic obstructive pulmonary disease:

- A male sex
- B homozygous serum-protease inhibitor deficiency
- C working with cadmium
- D working with aniline dyes
- E low socio-economic status

22.15 The following drugs increase theophylline metabolism:

- A propranolol
- B rifampicin
- C allopurinol
- D phenytoin
- E phenobarbitone

22. Respiratory Disorders

22.16 Pneumonia

    A caused by *Streptococcus pneumoniae* is the most common community acquired infection
    B caused by atypical organisms accounts for 15-20% of cases
    C occurs in up to 5% of hospitalized patients
    D causes more deaths than asthma in those under 50 years of age
    E in the community is rarely caused by Gram-negative bacteria

22.17 The following statements about asbestosis are true:

    A the first signs of asbestosis usually occur 2 to 3 years following exposure
    B pleural plaques are the most common radiological sign of exposure to asbestos
    C following diagnosis, active treatment with chest physiotherapy is required
    D heavy exposure to asbestos is normally necessary to cause asbestosis
    E fine end-inspiratory crackles at the lung bases are a reliable sign of asbestosis

22.18 *Pneumocystis carinii*

    A in Africa is much less common than tuberculosis as an opportunistic pathogen in AIDS
    B typically causes bilateral lower lobe shadowing on chest radiography
    C can be excluded as a cause of pneumonia in the presence of a normal chest radiograph
    D can be reliably detected using serological antibody tests
    E usually requires transbronchial lung biopsy to achieve a diagnosis

22.19 The recognized side-effects of rifampicin include

    A potentiation of anticonvulsants
    B conjunctivitis
    C hepatitis
    D lengthening of the half-life of warfarin
    E acute renal failure

22. Respiratory Disorders

22.20 Pulmonary sarcoidosis

- A is found more commonly in Afro-Caribbeans than in North Europeans
- B rarely remits spontaneously
- C is rare in patients under 30
- D can be reliably diagnosed using the Siltzbach-Kveim test
- E should be treated by steroids in most cases

22.21 Cryptogenic fibrosing alveolitis

- A seldom causes death
- B usually presents in childhood
- C is unusual for a lung disorder in that finger clubbing is rare
- D may be improved by high dose prednisolone
- E is classified as an occupational disease

22.22 Progressive massive fibrosis

- A is characterized on radiography by increased diffuse shadowing of all lobes
- B characteristically affects lower lobes first
- C is often associated with emphysema
- D may develop a long while after a worker has stopped coalmining
- E is linked with rheumatoid arthritis to form Huntingdon's syndrome

22.23 The following statements about coalworker's pneumoconiosis (CP) are true:

- A CP is characterized by small rounded opacities on radiography
- B quartz mining has a tendency to produce profuse fibrosis
- C simple CP is not associated with clinically significant impairment of lung function
- D the risk of developing simple CP is unrelated to the dose of coal dust inhaled
- E CP is associated with an increased risk of lung cancer

22. Respiratory Disorders

22.24 Adult respiratory distress syndrome commonly causes the following features:

    A lobar pneumonia on chest radiography
    B an elevated pulmonary arterial wedge pressure
    C increased platelet count
    D increased fibrinogen degradation products
    E increased lung compliance

22.25 The following statements about mechanical ventilation are true:

    A mechanical ventilation commonly causes the cardiac output to fall
    B mechanical ventilation can be used for the therapeutic manipulation of PaO_2 levels to control cerebral blood flow
    C mixed venous blood to monitor the ventilator's performance is conventionally sampled from the pulmonary artery
    D positive end expiratory pressure ventilation commonly reduces venous return
    E a normal PaO_2 indicates satisfactory oxygen delivery to peripheral tissues

22.26 Lung cancer

    A causes deaths in the ratio 2:1 for men and women in the UK
    B is most prevalent among people aged over 70 years
    C is most commonly adenocarcinoma among smokers
    D has a clear genetic association
    E is associated with the level of urban pollution

22.27 The following statements about mediastinal masses are true:

    A most asymptomatic masses are malignant
    B up to 50% of symptomatic masses are malignant
    C biopsy by fine-needle aspiration is generally a helpful investigation
    D biopsy of the anterior mediastinum is easier than the posterior mediastinum
    E ideally, surgical biopsy of middle mediastinal masses is via the second intercostal space

22. Respiratory Disorders

22.28 The following statements about the cytology of pleural fluid are true:

   A lymphocytes predominate in the presence of an acute infection
   B large numbers of mesothelial cells are found following pulmonary infection
   C malignant mesothelial cells confirm the presence of a mesothelioma
   D multinucleated giant cells are found in rheumatoid disease
   E cholesterol crystals are diagnostic of hypercholesterolaemia

22.29 The following patients are suitable for lung transplantation:

   A patients under 45 years of age
   B patients diagnosed as needing lung transplantation with single-stem coronary heart disease but no ECG changes
   C patients requiring assisted ventilation
   D young patients with severe respiratory impairment following a road traffic accident
   E patients with end-stage respiratory disease unresponsive to medical therapy

22.30 The following conditions are associated with bronchiectasis:

   A tuberculosis
   B histoplasmosis
   C allergic aspergillosis
   D measles
   E pertussis

23. RHEUMATOLOGY

23.1 The characteristic pathological features of osteoarthritis include

    A cyst formation
    B synovial proliferation
    C trabecular collapse
    D hypertrophy of ligaments
    E turbid synovial fluid

23.2 Rheumatoid factors

    A cause rheumatoid arthritis
    B are found in patients without arthritis
    C are autoantibodies
    D can be produced locally in joints
    E disappear from the peripheral blood following successful treatment of rheumatoid arthritis

23.3 The recognized extra-articular features of rheumatoid arthritis include

    A diarrhoea
    B impotence
    C pancreatitis
    D depression
    E lymphadenopathy

23.4 Ankylosing spondylitis

    A is as prevalent as rheumatoid arthritis
    B is associated with HLA-B27
    C improves with exercise
    D affects men more than women in a ratio of 10:1
    E is most unlikely if the ESR is normal

23. Rheumatology

23.5 Reiter's syndrome

A follows about 1-2% of cases of infective dysentery
B has an incidence of 10:1 male to female
C can present with buccal ulceration
D is usually self-limiting
E is linked with HLA-B27

23.6 Pseudogout

A is another name for acute urate arthropathy
B is the most common cause of acute monoarthritis in middle aged adults
C affects the knee more commonly than other joints
D is an unlikely diagnosis in the presence of systemic symptoms, such as fever and confusion
E is self-limiting

23.7 The following facts about the treatment of children with arthritis are true:

A children tolerate non-aspirin non-steroidal anti-inflammatory drugs worse than adults
B high dose corticosteroids are contraindicated in the treatment of systemic disease
C intra-articular corticosteroids have a useful role in the treatment of incapacity caused by one or two joints
D intra-articular corticosteroids should be used with caution because they may cause cartilage damage
E methotrexate is contraindicated because it produces too many undesirable side-effects in children

23.8 The incidence of disease increases with age in the following conditions:

A polymyositis
B dermatomyositis
C scleroderma
D giant cell arteritis
E polymyalgia rheumatica

23. Rheumatology

23.9 The following statements about magnetic resonance imaging are true:

A contrast between different types of soft tissue is low
B there is no radiation hazard
C three-dimensional imaging is possible
D pacemakers are not a contraindication
E hydrogen protons are the key body particles involved in obtaining an image

23.10 The following side-effects are linked with non-steroidal anti-inflammatory drugs:

A hypokalaemia
B polycythaemia
C neutrophilia
D thrombocytopenia
E hypocalcaemia

23.11 The following drugs and side-effects are linked:

A methotrexate and hepatic disease
B azathioprine and eye toxicity
C antimalarial drugs and non-Hodgkin's lymphoma
D penicillamine and loss of taste
E corticosteroids and avascular necrosis

23.12 Stress fractures

A can be reliably diagnosed by standard radiographs
B show first radiological signs of healing 4-8 weeks post fracture
C are rare in the pelvis
D are rarely painful at the fracture site
E can be confirmed by bone scintography

23. Rheumatology

23.13 Gout

    A predominantly affects males
    B is usually, but not always, accompanied by elevated serum uric acid levels
    C is associated with high alcohol intake, due to the high purine content of alcoholic drinks
    D is closely associated with potassium-sparing diuretics
    E can cause renal impairment

23.14 The following conditions characteristically present as a monoarthritis:

    A Charcot's joint disease
    B hypertrophic pulmonary osteoarthropathy
    C amyloidosis
    D acromegaly
    E Behçet's disease

24. SEXUALLY TRANSMITTED DISEASES

24.1 Anaerobic vaginosis

    A is caused by *Trichomonas vaginalis* infection
    B is characterized by a lower than normal vaginal pH
    C is characterized by the presence of 'clue cells'
    D occurs only in sexually active women
    E is best treated by procaine penicillin

24.2 *Chlamydia trachomatis* **may be a causative agent in**

    A neonatal meningitis
    B prostatitis in young men
    C epididymitis
    D neonatal otitis media
    E perihepatitis in women

24.3 The following facts about genital warts are true:

    A the incubation period may be up to 9 weeks
    B most warts in children over 2 years are associated with sexual abuse
    C following treatment genital warts rarely recur spontaneously
    D the most common cause is the herpes simplex virus
    E in the last 10 years the incidence has risen faster in women than in men

24.4 Tertiary syphilis is characterized by

    A cranial nerve lesions
    B osteoporosis
    C gummatous lesions of the skin
    D aortitis
    E tabes dorsalis

24. Sexually Transmitted Diseases

24.5 The following epidemiological features are associated with an increased risk of pelvic inflammatory disease (PID):

A previous episode of PID
B current use of intrauterine device
C age over 25 years
D recent pregnancy
E first sexual intercourse at an early age

24.6 Lymphogranuloma venereum

A is caused by *Haemophilus ducreyi* infection
B is more common among homosexuals than heterosexuals
C has an incubation period of 2-6 days
D has a primary stage characterized by the development of lymphadenitis
E in pregnant women, is best treated with erythromycin

24.7 The signs of granuloma inguinale include

A inguinal lymphadenopathy
B urethral stenosis
C vaginal bleeding
D elephantiasis of the external genitalia
E painless papule

24.8 Primary genital herpes

A usually presents with multiple painful ulcers
B presents, on average, 4-5 weeks following exposure
C is usually accompanied by dysuria
D may be followed by recurrent attacks, usually related to sexual intercourse
E does not usually cause inguinal lymphadenopathy

24. Sexually Transmitted Diseases

24.9 Neonatal gonococcal infection

- A is usually acquired by vertical transmission from an infected mother
- B is usually diagnosed 1-2 months following delivery
- C causes ophthalmia
- D causes disseminated disease in most babies
- E causes permanent neural deafness in about 2% of cases

24.10 The features of osteomalacia include

- A distal myopathy
- B low serum alkaline phosphatase levels
- C Heberden's nodules on radiography
- D excess osteoid in bone biopsy
- E bone pain

24.11 Familial hypophosphataemic rickets

- A is a sex-linked recessive disorder
- B is more severe in boys than in girls
- C usually presents at 1-3 years of age
- D is treated by phosphate supplements with vitamin D
- E impairs bone growth and causes deformities

24.12 The following statements about bone are true:

- A the serum activity of alkaline phosphatase reflects the functional activity of osteoclasts
- B osteocytes are derived from osteoblasts
- C collagen is made of polypeptide chains
- D osteoblasts produce the enzyme acid phosphatase
- E osteoid is the unmineralized part of the bone matrix

24. Sexually Transmitted Diseases

24.13 Parathyroid hormone

- A is secreted by the parathyroid glands in response to pituitary parathyroid hormone releasing factor
- B acts directly on the kidney to increase tubular reabsorption of calcium
- C reduces skeletal calcium turnover
- D acts directly on the small intestine to increase absorption of calcium
- E is involved in the metabolism of vitamin D

ANSWERS AND TEACHING NOTES

1. ALCOHOL/DRUG MISUSE ANSWERS

1.1 D Ref: 62, 2536-7
Alcohol dependence syndrome is characterized by an increased tolerance to alcohol, relief or avoidance of withdrawal symptoms by further drinking, a subjective awareness of the compulsion to drink and a narrowing of the drinking repertoire.

1.2 B C D E Ref: 62, 2538-42
In the 1960s and 1970s alcohol consumption in most Western countries rose sharply. However, during the past decade consumption has fallen in some (e.g. France and Italy) and levelled off in others (e.g. UK, Irish Republic, Canada, former West Germany). Abstinence or minimal alcohol consumption should still be encouraged for pregnant women, but available evidence suggests that the dangers of maternal drinking during pregnancy (the fetal alcohol syndrome) appear to have been exaggerated and that alcohol is only a minor contributor to birth defects.

1.3 B C Ref: 62, 2538-42
Publicans, deck hands, bargemen, boatmen, ship's officers, hotel managers, fishermen, chefs, journalists, drivers' mates, winders, reelers are some of the groups most likely to die from liver cirrhosis. 10 years ago doctors had 300 per cent greater than average risk of dying from cirrhosis, but the most recent (1986) OPCS survey shows this figure has dropped to just 15%.

1.4 A B D E Ref: 62, 2543-7
Ethanol is a CNS depressant. In small doses it interferes with cortical processes, in large doses with medullary function. Ethanol is a peripheral vasodilator and may cause hypoglycaemia, especially in children. Lactic acidosis is a serious but uncommon complication of acute ethanol intoxication.

1.5 B C Ref: 62, 2543-7
Marked variations occur in the symptoms of alcohol withdrawal, even in the same patient from one alcohol withdrawal episode to the next. Sympathetic nervous system hyperactivity is characterized by sweating, tachycardia, hypertension and tremor. Dysrhythmias are

Answers : Cardiology

rare and are probably secondary to hypokalaemia, hypomagnesaemia and acid-base disturbances.

1.6   A D E   **Ref: 62,** 2562-7
The clinical features of cannabis intake include euphoria with drowsiness, distorted and heightened images, altered tactile sensations, tachycardia, hypertension and ataxia with visual and auditory hallucinations. Injections may produce nausea and vomiting within minutes and, after about an hour, profuse watery diarrhoea.

1.7   A B C E   **Ref: 62,** 2562-7
The peak age group for volatile substance abuse is 13-15 years, with boys outnumbering girls 4:1. Abuse usually lasts less than 6 months, but about 10% of abusers become dependent and some will progress to illicit drugs and alcohol.

2. CARDIOLOGY ANSWERS

2.1   A C D   **Ref: 66,** 2720-5
Following myocardial infarction (MI) ventricular fibrillation is most likely to occur within the first few hours and is one of the more easily correctable causes of early death. The ECG can remain normal following even an extensive MI. Thrombolytic therapy, when indicated, should be started early and is not dependent on resolution of chest pain.

2.2   B C E   **Ref: 66,** 2725-31
Ejection systolic murmurs (ESM) are associated with aortic stenosis and are usually harsh, radiating to the neck. Atrial septal defects, not ventricular septal defects, cause ESM and their severity is directly proportional to the length of the murmur - the longer the murmur, the more severe the defect. However, should left ventricular failure intervene, the murmur may shorten and such patients may die very quickly. Mitral regurgitation is diagnosed by a diastolic murmur, not a systolic one. Aortic sclerosis can be difficult to differentiate from aortic stenosis. A short murmur with a clear second sound and a normally rising pulse suggests sclerosis.

Answers : Cardiology

2.3 B C   Ref: 66, 2725-31
Thyrotoxicosis is linked with rapid atrial fibrillation. Down's syndrome is linked with ventricular septal defect or patent ductus arteriosus, and Marfan's with aortic incompetence and ventricular or atrial septal defect.

2.4 D E   Ref: 66, 2732-8
Cardiomegaly exists when the cardiothoracic ratio is greater than 0.5 (i.e. the heart measures more than half the transthoracic diameter). Pressure overload produces ventricular hypertrophy rather than dilatation and the heart often remains normal or only slightly increased in size. Acute myocardial infarction rarely causes cardiomegaly although myocardial failure will. Mitral regurgitation is more likely to cause cardiomegaly than mitral stenosis.

2.5 A C D   Ref: 66, 2739-45
Inversion of the T wave in V1-V3 in a patient with chest pain suggests pulmonary embolism rather than myocardial infarction. Abnormalities of the T wave in lateral leads are not characteristic of digoxin toxicity which is more characterized by rhythm abnormalities, especially atrial and ventricular fibrillation.

2.6 C D   Ref: 66, 2761-7
The left atrium is the most difficult chamber to enter. Pressure measurements in the left ventricle are made via a catheter advanced against the blood flow through the femoral or brachial artery. A gradient of 70 mm Hg across the aortic valve indicates severe stenosis, though there is no definite value of valve gradient which indicates a need for surgery, the decision depends upon individual circumstances.

2.7 A B E   Ref: 67, 2768-9
Cigarettes, alcohol and caffeine are well accepted factors predisposing to palpitations. Heavy meals and a tendency to gastro-oesophageal reflux will also precipitate palpitations.

2.8 B C D E   Ref: 67, 2785-90
Digoxin and bethanidine both depress sinus node function to some extent in most people. Verapamil and many other anti-arrhythmic agents may cause difficulties in patients predisposed to sinus node dysfunction.

Answers : Cardiology

2.9 C   **Ref: 67, 2791-5**

The patient with acute heart failure should be placed in a sitting position and oxygen should be administered. Morphine reduces anxiety and diminishes reflex sympathetic activity thereby having a vasodilator effect. Digoxin has no place in the immediate treatment of a patient with acute heart failure. Nitrates have an immediate beneficial effect on the heart and may replace more traditional treatments of heart failure.

2.10 A C E   **Ref: 67, 2791-5**

Vasodilators increase cardiac output but lower left atrial pressure. They modify haemodynamics acutely but not long-term. This lack of chronic response may be due to development of tolerance, down-regulation of drug receptors, altered drug metabolism, neuro-humoral reactions or myocardial deterioration.

2.11 B D   **Ref: 67, 2791-5**

Angiotensin converting enzyme inhibitors (ACEIs) increase renal perfusion. They can also exacerbate renal failure and raise the plasma potassium which is why they should not be used with potassium sparing diuretics. ACEIs have been shown to prolong survival in patients with severe heart failure. The dilemma is whether they should be used earlier in treatment than they currently are.

2.12 B E   **Ref: 67, 2796-802**

In most patients with dilated cardiomyopathy the systolic blood pressure is low to normal. Coronary arteriography is necessary to exclude anomalous left coronary artery and coronary artery disease. Calcium antagonists are inappropriate therapy because they have a negative inotropic effect.

2.13 A   **Ref: 67, 2802-6**

Most aneurysms occur in the antero-apical and lateral regions of the left ventricle and are caused by occlusion of the anterior descending coronary artery. The 5-year survival for people with aneurysms varies between 10% and 20%. Although 22-50% of aneurysms contain laminated clots, systemic emboli are rare. Congestive heart failure is one of the indications for surgery.

Answers : Cardiology

2.14 B C D Ref: 67, 2802-6
Rupture of an interventricular septum causes a new pansystolic murmur which may also arise from mitral regurgitation since the two conditions may often co-exist. There is no particular reason why a ruptured septum should cause palpitations.

2.15 A C D E Ref: 68, 2818-23
Age is an important factor in deciding the outcome of an infarct. For example, one study conducted at a District General Hospital showed twice the mortality (30%) for patients over 65 years compared with patients under 65 years (15%). Low blood pressure is a poor prognostic feature in the post-infarction phase.

2.16 All false Ref: 68, 2830-3
Nitrates cause venous dilatation and therefore a reduction in venous return and cardiac output. Many nitrates give relief from angina for as long as an hour. Some nitrates (e.g. isosorbide dinitrate) are subject to first-pass liver metabolism.

2.17 E Ref: 68, 2834-6
The left main stem is not suitable for angioplasty because occlusion during attempted angioplasty might be catastrophic. Multiple vessel angioplasty is now commonplace. Previous bypass surgery is not a contraindication to angioplasty which may offer fewer risks than repeat surgery. The treatment of unstable angina may account for 25-30% of procedures in some centres.

2.18 B C D E Ref: 68, 2834-6
In experienced hands complications from coronary angiography are rare. Overall the mortality is about 0.2%. However they do increase with the severity of patients' symptoms, particularly poor left ventricular function, stenosis of the stem of the left coronary artery or widespread coronary artery disease.

2.19 A C D Ref: 68, 2837-44
Anti-arrhythmic drugs are not routinely recommended following myocardial infarction. They may not be effective against ventricular infarction. They may not be effective against ventricular fibrillation and some can induce arrhythmias themselves. β-blockers undoubtedly reduce fatality, although appropriate dosage is in doubt

Answers : Cardiology

for some. The simplest to use is timolol 5 mg b.d. increasing to 10 mg b.d. for a maximum of two years. Aspirin in the dose 150-160 mg/day is beneficial.

2.20 C D E   **Ref: 68,** 2848-54

The enzyme rise following myocardial infarction is due to leakage of intracellular enzymes out of infarcted myocardium into the bloodstream. Creatinine kinase (CK) is the first cardiac enzyme to rise following infarction. Peak lactate dehydrogenase or hydroxybutyrate dehydrogenase levels (not aspartate aminotransferase levels) give a crude estimate of infarct size.

2.21 A B C   **Ref: 69,** 2856-9

Concordance of blood pressure levels exists between siblings, non-identical twins and particularly identical twins. It can be shown between parents and children as young as 4-5 days old.

2.22 C D E   **Ref: 69,** 2884-7

Clinical examination of pericardial effusion will reveal increased cardiac dullness on auscultation and an apex beat which is difficult to palpate. There will be low blood pressure (and cardiac output) and low pulse pressure. Pulsus paradoxus occurs when the systolic blood pressure falls by 10 mm Hg or more on inspiration.

2.23 E   **Ref: 69,** 2864-71

If postural hypertension is suspected, pressure measurement should be taken standing. In pregnant women the blood pressure should be taken in the sitting or left lateral position since in the lying position the pregnant uterus may restrict venous return and lower blood pressure. The bladder of the sphygometer cuff should cover at least 80% of the arm circumference, otherwise artificially high readings are found. Differences in blood pressure between a patient's two arms are often seen so, at the first consultation, measurements should be carried out on both sides.

2.24 A C E   **Ref: 69,** 2864-71

Thiazide diuretics are contraindicated in patients with glucose intolerance, but not calcium antagonists. Calcium antagonists (or β-blockers) are indicated for hypertensive patients with ischaemic heart disease.

Answers : Cardiology

2.25 A B D Ref: 69, 2872-6

Angioplasty can be repeated several times if necessary although the chances of success fall with each repeat. Fibrinolytic therapy combined with angioplasty is showing good results. Both morbidity and mortality for angioplasty are minimal.

2.26 A B D Ref: 69, 2856-9

Blood pressure is lower in young females than males but this situation reverses following the menopause. Studies show that the tendency for elevated blood pressure is present from an early stage of development. Blood pressure is low among those who consume little alcohol compared to those who consume heavily.

2.27 A D E Ref: 69, 2884-7

Chest auscultation in acute pericarditis may reveal a pericardial friction rub of which there are three typical components: systolic, early diastolic (during rapid filling) and presystolic (during atrial contraction). The ECG usually shows raised ST segments, especially leads 1 and 2. The chest radiograph is typically normal, unless there is an additional pericardial effusion.

2.28 A D E Ref: 69, 2872-6

Measurement of the resting arm:ankle (not thigh) Doppler pressure index is useful. In older people symptoms in the legs are unlikely to be due to arterial disease if the pressure index is over 0.8. 75% of patients with intermittent claudication find their symptoms remain static or even improve following presentation, particularly in the first two years. In the remaining 25% deterioration occurs.

2.29 B C D Ref: 70, 2893-6

Children with tetralogy of Fallot present with an ejection systolic murmur, maximum in the pulmonary area but heard all over the pericardium. Its intensity may diminish with increasing cyanosis because the pulmonary outflow is so narrow as to be almost atretric. Squatting compresses the femoral arteries, increases systemic pressure and thereby causes a higher pressure in the ventricles which forces more blood across the obstructed pulmonary outflow.

Answers : Cardiology

2.30 A C E Ref: 70, 2893-6
The detection of central cyanosis depends on both the proportion of desaturated haemoglobin in the blood and the haemoglobin concentration. Thus, an anaemic child may not appear as cyanosed as a child with a similar oxygen saturation and a normal haemoglobin level. Finger clubbing secondary to congenital heart disease does not appear until approximately 3 months of age.

2.31 B C D E Ref: 70, 2901-7
Large ventricular septal defects are poorly tolerated by infants. Presentation usually occurs in the first month of life, or subsequently, with heart failure and failure to thrive. Direct repair is the surgical treatment of choice. Pulmonary banding used to be used in early infancy but is now only used in complex cases.

2.32 B D E Ref: 70, 2901-7
Cardiac catheterization should be avoided in neonates if at all possible because there is a risk of serious deterioration. Coarctation is associated with upper body hypertension and high pulmonary pressure because of high pulmonary vascular tone and left sided heart failure. Re-opening the ductus arteriosus with a prostaglandin infusion increases pressure in the lower body segment and may lead to improvement.

2.33 A B C Ref: 70, 2916-22
A collapsing pulse with sharp upstroke and wide pulse pressure is pathognomic of aortic regurgitation. The manifestations of this sign include visible capillary pulsation in the fingers (Quincke's sign) and head bobbing (de Musset's sign). In aortic regurgitation the aortic second heart sound is usually inaudible. Hepatomegaly is a sign of right heart failure which is not usually a feature of aortic regurgitation.

2.34 B C E Ref: 70, 2916-22
Rheumatic fever, but not rheumatoid arthritis, is associated with mitral regurgitation. A left atrial myxoma interferes with valve closure. A ventricular septal defect will cause aortic but not mitral regurgitation. Marfan's syndrome is often associated with a 'floppy' and leaky valve.

2.35 C D E   Ref: 70, 2923-8
Left ventricular hypertrophy follows aortic stenosis so ECG changes suggestive of it are one of the indications for valvotomy. Other indications include a significant pressure drop across the aortic valve and the risk of sudden death.

3. CLINICAL PHARMACOLOGY ANSWERS

3.1 A B C D   Ref: 59, 2408-15
The main site of drug metabolism is the liver but other organs such as the kidney, gut or lung can metabolize drugs to some extent. Most drugs are metabolized by oxidation and conjugation but a few 'pro-drugs' (e.g. cyclosporin, enelapril, levodopa) have no biological activity and need metabolic activation.

3.2 B C E   Ref: 59, 2408-15
Most drug absorption takes place in the upper small bowel because of its massive surface area. Opiates slow drug absorption because they slow the rate of gastric emptying. Lipid soluble drugs are absorbed quickly by passive diffusion. Water soluble drugs are best taken on an empty stomach; lipid soluble ones with food.

3.3 All False   Ref: 59, 2419-24
Peak drug concentrations are usually reached 30-60 minutes after ingestion. There are plenty of examples where the oral route of drug administration is not the safest; for example in patients with hepatic cirrhosis the oral administration of highly extracted drugs such as chlormethiazole increases blood concentrations several folds compared with intravenous administration. Aspirin weakens the gastric mucosal barrier systemically so the problem of local mucosal irritation continues. The purpose of sublingual administration is to bypass first-time liver metabolism.

3.4 B D E   Ref: 59, 2425-9
There is no value in monitoring serum concentrations of drugs when there is no relationship between serum values and therapeutic effects. The major indications for serum drug concentration measurement include ineffective treatment, suspected toxicity, suspected poor

Answers : Clinical Pharmacology

compliance, drug interactions and drug-disease interactions in which the pharmacokinetics of the drug are changed by the condition itself.

3.5   B D E   Ref: 59, 2429-34
Methysergide is a 5-HT antagonist. Cimetidine is a histamine antagonist. Most receptors have an endogenous agonist, and an antagonist is a drug or endogenous substance which prevents the effect of this agonist. Some antagonists do not by themselves cause any effects by binding to receptors.

3.6   A D E   Ref: 59, 2435-41
Some drugs stimulate increased amounts of the drug metabolizing enzymes to be produced in the liver. This increased activity accelerates the metabolism of other drugs metabolised in the same way so that increased dosages may be necessary to prevent treatment failure. Drugs known to have this effect include the barbiturates, phenytoin, rifampicin and halothane.

3.7   D E   Ref: 59, 2435-41
Some drugs inhibit or prevent the metabolism of other drugs either by affecting the enzyme system (for example cimetidine binds to cytochrome P-450 to have this effect), or by competing successfully for a metabolic pathway. Such drugs include chlorpromazine, erythromycin, cimetidine, tricyclic antidepressants and phenylbutazone.

3.8   B D E   Ref: 59, 2441-6
Glomerular filtration falls in the elderly, which is particularly significant for drugs with a narrow therapeutic ratio such as digoxin, lithium and the aminoglycosides. The reduced liver flow causes reduced clearance of drugs which undergo extensive first-pass metabolism. The significance of the prolongation of the elimination half-life for lipophilic drugs in the elderly is that the elimination half-life alone is not an accurate measure of drug metabolizing capacity.

3.9   A C   Ref: 60, 2456-9
There is little evidence that therapeutic levels of glucocorticoids have any significant effect on the levels of circulating IgG or IgE (immunoglobulins that are central to the development of allergic

Answers : Clinical Pharmacology

disease). At high doses glucocorticoids have mineralocorticoid-like effects including sodium retention and hypokalaemia. Glucocorticoids can cause growth retardation with prolonged use. They are linked with osteoporosis, not osteopetrosis.

3.10 E   Ref: 60, 2459-68

Calcium blockers reduce myocardial work, increase myocardial blood flow and oxygen supply, and cause direct coronary arterial vasodilation. For these reasons they are often valuable in angina although their role as monotherapy in chronic stable angina is still controversial. They work by blocking the uptake of calcium (especially slow channel) into cardiac cells.

3.11 C D   Ref: 60, 2469-73

Muscle tremor and hypokalaemia are both recognized side-effects of B_2-agonists but not theophylline. Impaired learning ability and behavioural disturbances are well recognized in children on theophylline as is irritability in the babies of mothers taking the drug. Rapid intravenous injection of theophylline may cause acute hypotension, not hypertension.

3.12 C D E   Ref: 60, 2474-9

Warfarin inhibits the synthesis of active prothrombin and Factors VII, IX and X; it also inhibits the action of the enzyme vitamin K epoxic reductase which facilitates the reconstitution of hepatic stores of vitamin K. Heparin combines with a plasma protein, anti-thrombin III to inhibit thrombin and the activated coagulation Factors XII, XI, X and IX.

3.13 C   Ref: 60, 2480-4

Oral contraceptive steroids protect against benign breast disease, carcinoma of the uterus and ovary. The risk of venous thrombosis and pulmonary embolism is related to the oestrogen content of the combined contraceptive pill.

3.14 D E   Ref: 60, 2485-8

Sulphonamides are unsuitable because they may cause kernicterus (and haemolysis in patients with glucose-6-phosphate dehydrogenase deficiency); aspirin because it may cause Reye's syndrome and lithium because it may result in cardiovascular collapse.

Answers : Clinical Pharmacology

3.15 C   **Ref: 60, 2489-93**
Clindamycin is linked with pseudomembranous colitis, metoclopromide with acute dystonia, chloramphenicol with aplastic anaemia and methysergide with retroperitoneal fibrosis.

3.16 A B C D E   **Ref: 60, 2489-93**
Not only are adverse drug reactions responsible for 4% of all hospital admissions and occur in 10-20% of hospital inpatients but they also may be responsible for 1/1000 deaths on medical wards and may occur in up to 5% of patients in general practice. The reason why women are more commonly affected than men is not known.

3.17 A C D   **Ref: 101, 4221-8**
Malabsorption syndromes seldom affect drug absorption. Drug absorption may be affected by abnormalities of the gut, for example oedema caused by heart failure. Because the liver is the most important site of first-pass metabolism, liver disease may alter oral dosage requirements without altering intravenous requirements. The rate of clearance of a drug is the best measure of the rate at which it is being eliminated from the body.

3.18 A C D   **Ref: 101, 4229-34**
Since subcutaneous blood perfusion is poor, absorption from this area is generally slower than from muscle. Oesophageal transit time is affected by position and may be as much as 5 minutes for patients who swallow an aspirin sized tablet with a small volume of water and then lie supine.

3.19 ABDE   **Ref: 101, 4229-34**
The rectal route offers a useful alternative when oral administration is not feasible because of palatability, nausea or unconsciousness. The disadvantages include the small mucosal surface available for absorption and the possibility of poor drug retention due to leakage or defaecation.

3.20 D E   **Ref: 101, 4229-34**
The concurrent intake of food reduces the absorption of ampicillin, captopril and tetracycline as well as other drugs such as melphalan and rifampicin. The type of food may be important. For example milk

reduces the gastrointestinal absorption of tetracycline whereas grapefruit increases the bioavailability of felodipine.

3.21 C D   Ref: 101, 4241-4
Atenolol is a selective β-receptor blocker. Minoxidil is a rarely used hypotensive agent which reduces vascular calcium concentrations by opening cell membrane ATP-dependent calcium channels. Nifedipine relieves angina and hypertension by opposing vascular spasm in large vessels and reducing resistance in small vessels. It is a calcium channel blocker.

3.22 B E   Ref: 101, 4244-8
Ethosuximide serum concentration is linearly related to dose so therapeutic drug monitoring (TDM) is unnecessary. TDM is indispensible for prescribing variation lithium clearance and the safe dose range is narrow. The threshold concentrations of seizure control and toxicity vary considerably in patients treated with sodium valproate so monitoring is not helpful. Primidone is a prodrug which is metabolized to its active derivatives phenobarbitone and phenylethylmalonamide. Phenytoin has a low therapeutic index and a narrow target range so effective prescription cannot be achieved without TDM.

3.23 D   Ref: 101, 4255-8
Stilboestrol is linked with vaginal carcinoma in female offspring. Halothane is linked with jaundice. Isoprenaline is linked with sudden cardiac arrhythmias rather than acute dystonia which is a characteristic adverse reaction of metoclopramide. Chloramphenicol may cause aplastic anaemia rather than pseudomembranous colitis which is, more typically, caused by clindamycin.

4. CRITICAL CARE ANSWERS

4.1 A B C D E   Ref: 71, 2937-40
An inspiratory:expiratory ratio of 1:2 is satisfactory for most patients, adding a short pause without gas flow at the end of inspiration. Mechanical ventilation increases intrathoracic pressure and therefore impedes cardiac filling and lowers cardiac output. For left ventricular failure it is advantageous because it ensures good ventilation, removes

Answers : Critical Care

the effort of breathing and effectively enhances systemic blood flow. Mechanical ventilation can be hazardous for patients with asthma because it increases the chances of pneumothorax and acute right heart failure.

4.2 B E   Ref: 71, 2940-3
It is usually necessary to start antimicrobial therapy before a focus of infection has been found. Imipenum and cilastatin is one popular regime, others prefer the combination of a penicillin, an aminoglycoside and metronidazole. Sucralfate provides protection against stress ulceration.

4.3 A B D E   Ref: 71, 2940-3
Alcoholism and uraemia predispose to sepsis because they impair an individual's immune function. Malnutrition rather than obesity predisposes to sepsis. Antacid therapy predisposes to pathogenic colonization of the gut and nasotracheal tubes disrupt host defence mechanisms.

4.4 A B C E   Ref: 71, 2944-7
Pre-eclampsia is associated with adult respiratory syndrome (ARDS) as is another complication of pregnancy - amniotic fluid embolism. About one third of patients with acute pancreatitis die from pulmonary complications, while respiratory insufficiency contributes to death in another one third. Cerebral oedema and intracranial haemorrhage are two causes of raised intracranial pressure which can lead to ARDS. The greatest experience of ARDS and oxygen toxicity comes from diving accidents.

4.5 B C E   Ref: 71, 2958-60
The opioids produce euphoria, drowsiness and analgesia but also nausea, decreased gastrointestinal motility and truncal rigidity. Impaired liver function increases the elimination half-life for morphine, as does impaired renal function.

4.6 A E   Ref: 71, 2964-7
The heart, following drowning, is 'irritable' and particularly prone to ventricular fibrillation at temperatures in the 28-32°C range. However, the routine use of antiarrhythmics is not advisable and the irritability passes with warming. It is now clear that barbiturates offer

Answers : Dermatology

little benefit in terms of neuronal protection and have the additional disadvantage of impairing white blood cell function. Steroids are no longer used for wet lung syndrome and may also impair normal immune function.

4.7   A D E   **Ref: 71,** 2968-74
Ventricular fibrillation should be treated by DC cardioversion up to a maximum of 320 J of delivered energy. Bretylium tosylate has better anti-fibrillatory properties than most other anti-arrhythmic agents. Adrenaline improves coronary and cerebral circulation and is now recommended before lignocaine.

4.8   B C E   **Ref: 71,** 2968-74
Dopamine is an inotropic agent useful for treating the failing heart but has no role in ventricular tachycardia. Mysoline is indicated in the management of grand mal epilepsy.

5. DERMATOLOGY ANSWERS

5.1   D E   **Ref: 102,** 4264
Cicatrice is a scar; keratosis is the horny thickening. Papule is a small, superficial elevation of up to 1 cm in diameter, while macule is discoloured skin. The characteristic of erythema is that it does blanche on pressure, in contrast to purpura which does not.

5.2   A D   **Ref: 102,** 4273-7
Lithium has been reported as both precipitating and exacerbating psoriasis. Hydralazine has been linked with a number of conditions, for example systemic lupus erythematosis, but not psoriasis. β-blockers may act as both exacerbator and precipitant of psoriasis.

5.3   B E   **Ref: 102,** 4273-7
Oral contraceptives are characteristically linked with melasma, a brownish pigmentation on the face. Both codeine and aspirin can cause urticaria. Exfoliative dermatitis is usually caused by carbamazepine, allopurinol, gold, phenytoin, captopril or diltiazem but not tetracycline. Fucidin usually causes eczema rather than pigmentation.

Answers : Dermatology

5.4 B C E Ref: 102, 4278-81
Herpes simplex is usually associated with erythema multiforme. The infections associated with erythema nodosum include tuberculosis, leprosy and coccidiomycosis. Hyperthyroidism usually causes pruritus or urticaria rather than erythema nodosum. Most rheumatic diseases are associated with erythema nodosum including Behçet's disease.

5.5 B C E Ref: 102, 4285-8
The condition of most patients with atopic eczema improves during pregnancy. However some patients suffer deterioration which may be caused by increased excoriation from pruritus gravidarum. Hidradenitis suppurativa also usually improves during pregnancy.

5.6 D E Ref: 102, 4289-92
Milia are keratin cysts which appear shortly after birth and have no connection with tuberous sclerosis. Mongolian patches are congenital macular slate-grey or black patches, most commonly appearing in Afro-Caribbean and oriental babies. Port wine stains are present at birth and consist of irregularly dilated mature endothelial-lined capillary vessels confined to the upper dermis. They may occur in Sturge-Weber syndrome.

5.7 A E Ref: 102, 4298-301
Infantile atopic dermatitis usually starts on the cheeks and spreads to most parts of the body although the nappy area is generally spared. The flexor surfaces of limbs are usually involved in adult atopic dermatitis. The evidence that breast-feeding prevents atopic dermatitis is pretty thin; however breast-feeding should be encouraged for its general benefits.

5.8 B D E Ref: 103, 4304-7
Rosacea is characterized by pustules. Pimples sparing the vermillion border are characteristic of perioral dermatitis. The facial eruption of carcinoid syndrome is usually plum or purple coloured lasting about 20 minutes.

5.9 A B C E Ref: 103, 4308-11
Decreased nutritional supply to the nail matrix leads to a defective band of nail formation, resulting in a transverse groove made of thinner

Answers : Dermatology

nail plate. Since fingernails grow at about 1 mm/week it is possible to date previous illnesses. The other major cause of these grooves is psoriasis. Opacity of the nail is suggestive of diabetes mellitus, cardiac failure and psoriasis. Blue nails are found as a side-effect of anti-malarial drugs such as chloroquine; whereas green nails are caused by *Pseudomonas* spp.

5.10 A D   Ref: 103, 4316-21
Cholestatic pruritus may be improved by drugs which speed hepatic microsomal function (such as phenobarbitone). Pruritus is reported in as few as 1% of diabetics. Iron deficiency (rather than folate deficiency) may cause pruritus which in turn responds to iron therapy.

5.11 A B C E   Ref: 103, 4322-7
Congenital melanocytic naevi are large, deeply pigmented lesions, present at birth. The risk of malignancy appears higher in large (over 5 cm diameter) naevi. Dysplastic naevi are large, active, mainly truncal naevi which occur in adults and may be solitary or multiple. There is an increased risk of melanoma in people with these lesions.

5.12 A E   Ref: 103, 4328-30
Basal cell carcinoma (BCC) does sometimes occur on covered skin sites for reasons unknown. Ultraviolet light is probably a tumour promoter rather than an initiator. The characteristic BCC cell is large but contains a heavily stained nucleus and no cytoplasm. Curettage and cautery in skilled hands remain a perfectly acceptable means of treatment.

5.13 All False   Ref: 103, 4328-30
There is no link between Bowen's disease and sun. Covered sites on the legs and trunk may be involved in Bowen's disease. There is no link with internal malignancy and the lesion only rarely metastasises. Bowen's disease occurs within the epidermis of skin where there is parakeratosis and acanthosis. Histologically the dermo-epidermal junction is retained, but if breached, indicates squamous cell carcinoma.

Answers : Diabetes

5.14 B C   Ref: 103, 4331-3
Dermatophyte infection (DI) is a major cause of alopecia worldwide. No link between DI and cancer has been demonstrated, and it is not a presenting feature of dermatomyositis.

5.15 B C   Ref: 103, 4340-3
In 60% of teenagers acne will be of sufficient severity for them to treat themselves with proprietary preparations or seek medical advice. Circulating levels of androgen are usually normal in patients with acne. The blackhead is caused by the plug within the pilosebaceous duct expanding to dilate the pilosebaceous orifice and gradually become extruded.

6. DIABETES ANSWERS

6.1 A E   Ref: 65, 2684-9
Non-insulin dependent diabetes (NIDDM) adversely affects both length and quality of life due to serious complications. The reduction in life expectancy averages 5-10 years in middle-aged patients with NIDDM. Macrovascular complications are frequently observed, regardless of age at diagnosis. Most patients demonstrate resistance to insulin action and may have high fasting levels although these are still lower than would be found in weight-matched normal subjects with similar plasma glucose levels.

6.2 All false   Ref: 65, 2689-92
The modern diabetic diet need not be markedly different from that eaten by a health conscious family. Diet is the mainstay of management of non-insulin dependent diabetes but it also plays a crucial role in the management of insulin dependent diabetes. Fat should represent 30% of the total energy intake, mainly in the unsaturated form. The recommendation for a low carbohydrate diet has now changed and been replaced with a diet in which carbohydrates provide 50-60% total energy provided the diet is also high in fibre, especially soluble fibre.

6.3 B C E   Ref: 65, 2695-9
Arterio-venous nipping and papilloedema are characteristic of hypertensive retinopathy.

Answers : Endocrine Disorders

6.4 A C D Ref: 65, 2700-3
Tinel's sign is used to diagnose the entrapment neuropathy, carpal tunnel syndrome. Reflexes do not form part of the autonomic system.

6.5 A B D Ref: 65, 2704-5
Renal biopsy for diabetic nephropathy is not routinely indicated. It is only necessary if nephrotic syndrome or de novo renal failure develops rapidly, or when retinopathy is absent. Tight control of diabetes does not significantly alter the cause of established disease, nor is it yet clear whether it can avert the development of nephropathy even if applied very early on in the disease.

6.6 A B C Ref: 65, 2713-6
Urinary ketones can be absent during diabetic ketoacidosis if the major increase is in α-hydroxybutyrate rather than acetoacetate. Hyperglycaemia is the rule. Creatinine levels may be falsely raised because ketoacids interfere with some assays.

6.7 A B C D Ref: 65, 2713-6
Infection is a common precipitant of diabetic ketoacidosis. Other precipitants include failure to increase or even maintain insulin therapy following myocardial infection, stroke and trauma or unnoticed interruption of insulin delivery in diabetics treated with continuous subcutaneous insulin infusion. Mortality without treatment is almost invariable.

7. ENDOCRINE DISORDERS ANSWERS

7.1 C E Ref: 63, 2576-82
Growth hormone levels are not suppressed normally following an oral glucose load in acromegalics. About 25% of acromegalics have impaired glucose tolerance. About 75% of acromegalics have a reduction in growth hormone levels following treatment with bromocriptine but this treatment should be regarded as an adjunct to surgery and/or radiotherapy.

7.2 A C D Ref: 63, 2588-95
Graves' disease is an immunologically mediated form of hyperthyroidism. Signs ACD are usually present but one or more may

Answers : Endocrine Disorders

be absent, for example elderly people may not have a detectable goitre. Ophthalmopathy is present in 50% of patients when first seen but may also develop after successful treatment or even before the development of hyperthyroidism.

7.3 C D E Ref: 63, 2596-600

Hypothyroidism is usually treated with T4, starting therapy slowly (e.g. 50 µg/day). Primary hypothyroidism is more common than the secondary hypothyroidism due to failure of TSH secretion.

7.4 B C E Ref: 63, 2601-4

Papillary thyroid carcinoma is usually multifocal, spreads locally but very rarely to lungs or bones. A few patients are managed by ipsilateral total lobectomy and isthmusectomy but most undergo a bilateral lobectomy. In the past, radioiodine ablation has been commonly used but probably should be confined to patients at risk of tumour recurrence.

7.5 All False Ref: 63, 2611-15

A recent survey of 1 million Londoners revealed only 39 had Addison's disease, so it is uncommon. Thomas Addison (1795-1860) was a British physician. Plasma ACTH is high due to loss of negative feedback by circulating cortisol. The short tetracosactrin (Synacthen) test is usually performed for diagnostic purposes. There is no good evidence that pregnancy is contraindicated and even steroid replacement doses need not be changed except in special circumstances (e.g. toxaemia).

7.6 B C D E Ref: 63, 2616-20

Vasopressin is synthesized mainly in the supraoptic and paraventricular nuclei of the hypothalamus from where it migrates to the posterior pituitary. Vasopressin secretion is suppressed when plasma osmolality falls below 280 mosmol/kg. The action of splanchnic vasoconstriction is the reason why vasopressin is sometimes given to control gastrointestinal bleeding.

7.7 A B C Ref: 63, 2620-3

Tricyclic antidepressants may cause this syndrome but not MAO1 antidepressants. Inappropriate antidiuresis is not a recognized complication of carbidopa.

Answers : Endocrine Disorders

7.8 C D E   Ref: 64, 2624-31

Reliable radioimmunoassay tests for parathyroid hormone (PTH) are now widely available. The stimulus for synthesis and release of PTH is hypocalcaemia.

7.9 A B C E   Ref: 64, 2638-43

Pituitary causes of delayed puberty include tumours, sarcoidosis, tuberculosis, haemochromatosis, and histiocytosis X. Gonadal causes include testicular ageneas, testicular torsion, Klinefelter's, Turner's and Noonan's syndromes and XX or XY gonadal dysgenesis.

7.10 A D   Ref: 64, 2643-6

Inhibin is a glycoprotein hormone with a negative feedback effect (with testosterone) on FSH levels; it is secreted by Sertoli cells of the seminiferous tubules following FSH stimulation. Testosterone is produced by Leydig cells following stimulation by LH and has a negative feedback effect on LH not gonadotrophin releasing hormone.

7.11 A C D   Ref: 64, 2647-9

Gynaecomastia occurs in neonates as a result of transplacental transfer of high levels of maternal oestrogens into the baby's bloodstream at term. Decreased androgen production often results in gynaecomastia whether it is hypergonadotrophic (e.g. Klinefelter's syndrome, castration or orchitis) or hypogonadotrophic. Gynaecomastia is a recognized complication of drugs such as digitalis, spironolactone and cimetidine but not methyldopa.

7.12 C E   Ref: 64, 2656-9

The classical hormonal findings in polycystic ovary syndrome include high serum LH levels and low serum FSH levels. There may also be high androgen and oestradiol levels. The cause may be defective synthesis in the ovaries of oestradiol resulting in overproduction of precursors which may be metabolised in extraglandular tissue to oestrone and testosterone. Laparoscopy will reveal the characteristic appearance of the ovaries.

7.13 B C   Ref: 64, 2660-3

The menopause is accompanied by a depletion of ovarian oocytes accompanied by a fall in oestrogen production which causes a rise in pituitary hormones, LH and FSH. Osteoclasts are responsible for bone resorption (not formation) and their activity is accelerated by the menopause, for reasons not understood. Calcium supplements appear to have a minor effect on cortical bone loss and no effect on trabecular bone, where osteoporosis is most likely to occur.

7.14　All False　　　　　　Ref: 64, 2664-9
Since endocrine hypertension accounts for only 1-5% of all cases of hypertension it is neither practical nor economical to subject every patient with hypertension to full endocrine screening. The WHO definition of hypertension is any blood pressure greater than 160/95 mm Hg. Oestrogens, not testosterone, are the most common cause of endocrine hypertension in the developed world. Thus the progesterone-only pill is the least likely contraceptive pill to cause hypertension.

8. GASTROENTEROLOGY ANSWERS

8.1　A B　　　　　　Ref: 77, 3182-7
There is no evidence at the moment to prove a causal relationship between non-steroidal anti-inflammatory drugs and duodenal ulceration. Recent trial data shows that duodenal ulceration is often a chronic disease with frequent relapses. Duodenal ulceration causes epigastric pain some hours after a meal, when the patient is hungry.

8.2　D　　　　　　Ref: 77, 3182-7
Benign gastric ulceration occurs most commonly on the lesser curve of the stomach. Ulcers often penetrate into the muscularis mucosa. Patients with gastric ulcers secrete normal or subnormal amounts of gastric juice. It is impossible to distinguish between gastric and duodenal ulcer pain from the history.

8.3　A B C D　　　　　　Ref: 77, 3188-93
Pyoderma gangrenosum (as well as erythema nodosum) is linked to inflammatory bowel disease and bleeding disorders would be characterized by petechiae or purpura.

Answers : Gastroenterology

8.4 E Ref: 77, 3188-93

The mortality from acute upper gastrointestinal haemorrhage is 10%, rising in elderly patients. The most common cause (30%) is peptic ulcer disease. The association between acute upper gastrointestinal bleeds and steroid therapy is unclear. Haemoglobin estimation is a poor guide to the degree of acute bleeding because haemodilution takes place several hours later. Stress ulcers causing severe gastrointestinal bleeding are a recognized complication of severe burns and overwhelming sepsis.

8.5 C D Ref: 77, 3194-8

In the USA, gastric adenocarcinoma is the eighth major cause of death from cancer, but there has been a marked decrease in incidence overall. The tumour is about three times more common in the lowest socio-economic groups compared with the highest. Japanese mortality for gastric adenocarcinoma is about 70/100,000. Radiotherapy has little or no role in the treatment of gastric adenocarcinoma.

8.6 A B D E Ref: 77, 3194-8

Diet may well be important in the aetiology of gastric cancer. A high salt intake and living in areas with a high nitrate content in the soil seem to be aetiological factors. Iodine is associated with thyroid disorders, not gastric cancer. In addition to exposure to rubber processing, aflatoxins and nickel refining appear to be risk factors. Chronic gastritis, particularly type A, is associated with gastric adenocarcinoma.

8.7 E Ref: 77, 3204-9

Double-contrast barium meal coats the gastric mucosa with high density, concentrated barium while the lumen is filled with gas to produce the 'double-contrast' effect. It requires prior fasting for at least 6 hours to ensure the stomach is empty and is less operator-dependent than single-contrast meals. Constipation following the procedure is common and can be prevented by a high fluid intake and laxatives.

8.8 A B D Ref: 78, 3216-21

Patients with coeliac disease respond to a gluten-free diet, not a gluten diet. There is an increased risk of gastrointestinal cancer, especially

Answers : Gastroenterology

colon and oesophagus, associated with coeliac disease. The associated skin condition is dermatitis herpetiformis.

8.9 C E   Ref: 78, 3216-21
The link between lactose intolerance (LI) and osteoporosis is not established, particularly as LI occurs most commonly in people living in sunny climates where osteoporosis is generally not a problem. LI is unusual in northern Europeans. LI is demonstrated by low levels of jejunal lactase.

8.10 C E   Ref: 78, 3222-6
The xylose absorption test is abnormal. The Schilling test reveals B12 malabsorption due to ileal pathology, more severe than that of gluten enteropathy. Jejunal biopsy shows blunting but not flattening of villi.

8.11 A B C D E   Ref: 78, 3226-30
Up to 10% of infants and young children with cystic fibrosis (CF) develop rectal prolapse. Malnutrition and steatorrhoea may contribute to the genesis of this problem but it can occur in the absence of other symptoms so all children with rectal prolapse should be investigated for CF. The cirrhosis of CF occurs as focal biliary cirrhosis and multilobular biliary cirrhosis. Portal hypertension complicates 10% of older CF patients.

8.12 A B   Ref: 78, 3236-42
The incidence of pancreatic cancer has doubled in the last 50 years, particularly affecting males of African and Maori extraction. Pancreatic cancer is usually an adenocarcinoma, occurring most commonly in the head of the pancreas (70%). Tumour-specific antigen is an unreliable diagnostic investigation.

8.13 A   Ref: 78, 3236-42
One survey of autopsies in a hospital with an interest in pancreatitis revealed a large number of patients had died of undiagnosed acute pancreatitis (of whom only 10% had complained of abdominal pain). Alcohol and gallstones are common aetiological factors but the idiopathic form is the most common. Diagnosis of pancreatitis occurs once the serum amylase level is five times the upper limit of normal. ERCP can be safely used for the investigation of acute pancreatitis provided the operator is expert.

Answers : Gastroenterology

8.14 A B D E   Ref: 78, 3243-7

As a result of the wasting of bile there is a reduction in the concentration of bile salts in the bile in relation to cholesterol and phospholipids which predisposes to the formation of gallstones. Hyperoxaluria is a complication of steatorrhoea which predisposes to renal stones. Metabolic acidosis (not alkalosis) complicates short bowel syndrome because of lactic acidosis due to excessive absorption of D-lactic acid from the colon. Short bowels may not be able to metabolize amino acids by bacteria depriving the body of essential nutrients and causing hypoproteinuria.

8.15 A   Ref: 78, 3248-54

Acute appendicitis can occur at any age but is uncommon in children and elderly people. About 75% of patients have a WBC over 12,000 mm but in the remainder the count is normal or only marginally raised. Appendicitis is not associated with any specific bacteria or virus. Radiographs can exclude conditions which mimic appendicitis (e.g. a right uretic calculus) but are not diagnostic.

8.16 A B C E   Ref: 79, 3259-63

Cimetidine causes diarrhoea rather than constipation. Both tricyclics and monoamine oxidase inhibitors may cause constipation. Iron most commonly causes constipation but it can also cause diarrhoea.

8.17 A E   Ref: 79, 3263-8

Dyspareunia and urinary frequency affect approximately 42% and 61% respectively of patients with irritable bowel syndrome.

8.18 A   Ref: 79, 3263-8

Irritable bowel syndrome (IBS) most commonly presents in the mid-thirties: patients are seldom over 50 years. Symptoms of IBS are common in childhood and many adults with IBS give a history which extends back to childhood.

8.19 A C E   Ref: 79, 3275-9

Ileal disease associated with an abdominal mass and malabsorption is common in Crohn's disease. Bloody diarrhoea associated with colonic disease occurs in Crohn's disease but is more common in ulcerative colitis. Aphthoid ulceration is often the first sign of Crohn's disease. Mucin glands are usually preserved in Crohn's disease.

Answers : Gastroenterology

8.20 C D Ref: 79, 3275-9
Although a high intake of refined sugar and a low-fibre diet has been noticed in patients with Crohn's disease, a change of diet has no influence on the course of the disease. Crohn's disease is most common among northern Europeans and North Americans.

8.21 C Ref: 79, 3280-5
Gastrointestinal histoplasmosis is a fungal disease produced by *Histoplasma capsulatum*. It is prevalent in certain areas of the USA, but occurs in Europe as well. Complement fixation tests are positive in about 75% of cases but it is best diagnosed by biopsy of the affected area, when the organism may be demonstrated in histiocytes. It was invariably fatal prior to the introduction of amphotericin which is effective (and safer when given orally).

8.22 A B C E Ref: 79, 3286-91
Dermatitis may be due to the effects of the effluent on the skin or due to a contact dermatitis caused by an allergy to an adhesive or appliance. Renal calculi occur in 10% of male ileostomates in the UK. This is due to persistently high ileostomy losses causing a metabolic acidosis, and low urine volume. Cholesterol gallstones may occur as a result of the loss of the terminal ileum, thus interrupting the enterohepatic circulation of bile salts. Despite adaptation the volume of ileostomy effluent is greater than that of faeces, and ileostomates are particularly liable to salt and water depletion. Parastomal hernia is the most common complication.

8.23 D E Ref: 80, 3292-5
Colonoscopy with biopsy is the most accurate means of diagnosing and assessing inflammatory bowel disease; it should only be avoided in acute flare-ups. Colonoscopy is a valuable means of diagnosing, treating and following-up patients with colonic cancer. Profuse rectal bleeding may clear the bowel enabling an accurate diagnosis to be made.

8.24 A B E Ref: 80, 3300-4
The lifetime risk of developing colorectal cancer is 4%, the risk rising steeply with each decade after 40 years of age. The cost effectiveness and benefit of screening asymptomatic patients has not yet been

Answers : Gastroenterology

established. Abdominal palpation will detect approximately 10% of patients with colorectal cancer.

8.25 All False   **Ref: 80, 3305-7**
The sigmoid colon is supplied by the inferior mesenteric artery. Ischaemia particularly affects watershed areas of the bowel such as distal transverse colon, spheric flexure and rectosigmoid.

8.26 D   **Ref: 80, 3305-7**
Diverticular disease is the clinical syndrome which complicates diverticulosis, so by definition it cannot occur without symptoms. The sigmoid colon is the most commonly affected segment of the bowel to be affected by diverticular disease. Rectal bleeding seldom occurs, but when it does occur it usually settles spontaneously without treatment. The treatment for acute diverticular disease is hospitalization, rest, analgesia (avoiding morphine) and antibiotics including metronidazole. Surgery is rarely necessary acutely.

8.27 C D E   **Ref: 80, 3308-11**
Herpes simplex infection of the rectum is usually caused by type 2 virus. Important clinical features include inguinal lymphadenopathy, anorectal pain, constipation, perianal lesions, fever and neurological symptoms such as difficulty in initiating micturition. Oral acyclovir given within 6 days of the onset of a primary attack will reduce the severity, duration and incidence of complications and may be useful prophylactically for those with frequent relapses or who are immunocompromised.

8.28 A B E   **Ref: 80, 3321-6**
Carbohydrates (particularly refined sugars) should be avoided because they cause the reactive hypoglycaemia which is responsible for the symptoms of dumping syndrome. High fibre food should be encouraged because it slows the speed of gastric emptying and reduces the rate of carbohydrate absorption.

8.29 A B E   **Ref: 80, 3321-6**
Iron and B12 deficiency anaemias are recognized complications of gastric surgery but folate deficiency is not. Osteomalacia (but not osteoporosis) used to be a worrying complication of radical sub-total

9. GENETICS ANSWERS

9.1   **A B D E**   Ref: 58, 2376-80
Fetal tissue sampling is valuable in the diagnosis of some serious skin disorders and a small number of rare metabolic disorders. Chorionic villus sampling is particularly suitable for DNA diagnosis, particularly haemoglobinopathies, cystic fibrosis, X-linked muscular dystrophy, Huntington's chorea and the haemophilias. Serum α-fetoprotein is used for the diagnosis of neural tube defects and chromosome and other abnormalities. Detailed ultrasound examination will detect most cases of severe congenital heart disease.

9.2   **A B C D E**   Ref: 58, 2381-3
The normal human has 46 chromosomes, made up of 22 pairs of autosomes and one pair of sex chromosomes (XX in the female, XY in the male). Abnormalities may involve an alteration in the number of chromosomes (aneuploidy) or structural changes of one or more of the chromosomes. By term about 5% of still births and 0.5% of live births have an identifiable chromosome anomaly. Altogether there are as many as 50-100,000 genes.

9.3   **A C D E**   Ref: 58, 2385-9
No more than 3-5% of DNA codes for protein, most of the remainder has no known function. There are about 50,000 genes ranging in size from 1 kilobase to 2 megabases. Over 200 different restriction enzymes isolated from different species of bacteria have been described; they play a central role in molecular biological techniques.

9.4   **A B E**   Ref: 58, 2390-4
Duchenne muscular dystrophy affects boys. It is an incurable and tragic disease which usually kills affected children by the late teens. It is linked with the partial or complete absence of the muscle protein dystrophin. Dystrophin is a large protein but is present only in small amounts which explains why it has only recently been detected.

Answers : Haematology

9.5 D Ref: 58, 2395-7
Inheritance of Huntington's disease (HD) is autosomal dominant and the children of someone with HD will have a 50% chance of inheriting the disease. New mutations are very rare and a negative family history should always be carefully investigated. The HD gene has been localised, using DNA markers, to the short arm of chromosome 4.

9.6 B C E Ref: 58, 2397-9
Neurological disturbances in Wilson's disease are always of the motor system, except headache. Psychoses indistinguishable from schizophrenia or manic depression are well recognized. Kayser-Fleisher rings in Descemet's membrane of the cornea are characteristic.

9.7 B Ref: 58, 2399-406
Phenylketonuria is caused by an inborn deficiency of the hepatic enzyme phenylalanine hydroxylase activity. Impaired melanin production causes abnormally pale hair and eyes and the skin is prone to eczematous changes. Treatment is by a low phenylalanine, high tyrosine diet until about aged 12. Thereafter most experts lift dietary restrictions (except during pregnancy), but some recommend a diet low in protein rather than completely free. High levels of phenylalanine are toxic to a fetus causing microcephaly, mental retardation and congenital heart disease among other malformations.

10. HAEMATOLOGY ANSWERS

10.1 A D E Ref: 96, 3984-9
Differential white cell counts are accurate provided the cell morphology is normal. If it is not, careful visual inspection of the blood film is essential. The normal range for neutrophils tends to be lower in people of African origin than Europeans. Acute viral infections commonly cause neutropenia. Viral infections and pregnancy commonly reduce the platelet count.

10.2 D E Ref: 96, 3995-4002
Iron deficiency is linked with microcytic anaemia, as are vitamins A and C and pyridoxine deficiencies. Cobalamin deficiency is linked with megaloblastic anaemia, as is folic acid deficiency.

Answers : Haematology

10.3 A C D Ref: 96, 3995-4002
The main site of iron absorption is the duodenum. Haem iron, present in meat, is more readily absorbed than inorganic iron. Although inorganic iron usually predominates in the diet, relatively little can be made available for absorption, the exact amount depending on the presence or absence of dietary components and gastrointestinal secretions which enhance the solubility of iron.

10.4 A D E Ref: 96, 4003-5
Haemolytic states reduce the production of bilirubin. Bilirubin is transported from the reticuloendothelial system bound to plasma albumin (which prevents excretion by the kidney), is conjugated in the hepatic cells and then excreted into the bile. In the bowel bilirubin is converted to urobilinogen which is either excreted in the urine or reabsorbed by the gut and re-excreted in the bile. When haemoglobin is released into the circulation up to 200 mg/100 ml binds to haptoglobin and the complex is cleared. When this process happens more quickly than haptoglobin can be synthesised, the levels of serum haptoglobin fall. When the haptoglobin-binding capacity is exceeded free haemoglobin is degraded and the haem tends to bind to haemopexin or albumin forming methaemalbumin.

10.5 B D Ref: 96, 4005-11
Glucose-6-phosphate dehydrogenase deficiency (G-6-PD) is a common Y-linked trait thought to affect about 100 million people worldwide. Acute haemolysis follows ingestion of fava beans (not spices). The diagnosis is made by a simple assay for G-6-PD activity.

10.6 D E Ref: 96, 4012-5
It is the transplacental transfer of maternal antibodies which causes haemolytic anaemia of the newborn (HAN). HAN involving the ABO blood system accounts for 50% of all cases but is much less severe than that involving the Rhesus blood system. HAN due to ABO blood group incompatibility can occur without prior sensitization because anti-A and anti-B antibodies occur naturally.

10.7 A B D Ref: 97, 4035-8
Some antibiotics including chloramphenicol, penicillin, cephalosporins and sulphonamides (but not tetracycline) are linked with aplastic anaemia. Of the anti-inflammatory agents

Answers : Haematology

phenylbutazone, indomethacin, gold and penicillamine are linked but not diclofenac.

10.8 A B D E Ref: 97, 4038-44
Remission achieved within 4 weeks is a good prognostic indicator. Other good features include a white cell count less than 10×10^9/litre, age 2-10 years and female sex.

10.9 A B C E Ref: 97, 4038-44
Benzene and its derivatives are associated with acute leukaemia, as are the chromosomal disorders Down's syndrome and Fanconi's anaemia. Babies with Down's syndrome may develop a transient leukaemoid blood picture soon after birth, acute leukaemia may develop months or years later. The supposition is that trisomy 21 is a step in the leukaemogenic progess. Human lymphotrophic virus HTLV1 is associated with adult T cell leukaemia/lymphoma syndrome. The virus is endemic in Japan but occurs sporadically elsewhere, notably the West Indies.

10.10 B D E Ref: 97, 4045-9
The lymphocyte cell morphology and count is abnormal in chronic lymphocytic leukaemia (CLL). The immunoglobulins are usually low, occasionally a monoclonal band is present in urine or serum. Bone marrow aspiration and biopsy show infiltration by lymphocytes, useful as an indication of bone marrow reserves. Anaemia is usually present and it is important to distinguish between anaemia secondary to bone marrow failure and anaemia due to antoimmune haemolytic anaemia.

10.11 A B C Ref: 97, 4045-9
Anaemia is common, especially when the spleen is enlarged. The differential white count shows increased absolute numbers of the granulocyte series, particularly neutrophils and myelocytes, and basophilia is common. The platelet count is typically raised but can be low or normal. Serum vitamin B12 is usually very high due to increased transcobalamin 1 production.

10.12 D E Ref: 97, 4045-9
Chronic lymphocytic leukaemia (CLL) is usually caused by malignant transformation of a B cell, only 1% are caused by transformation in a T cell. CLL is hardly ever seen in the Orient, but is the most common

Answers : Immunology and AIDS

form seen in Europe and the USA. CLL usually occurs in people over 40. Chemotherapy for CLL is not curative so during the early stages many patients require no treatment. Only when the patient develops symptoms, symptomatic lymphadenopathy or autoimmune phenomena, should treatment begin.

10.13 D E **Ref: 97, 4058-61**
In myelodysplastic disorders the spleen is not enlarged, the blood count is usually low with no basophilia by contrast with myeloproliferative disorders in which splenomegaly, a high blood count and basophilia are present. The characteristic features of myelodysplastic disorders are the increased marrow cellularity and dysplasia.

10.14 A C E **Ref: 97, 4066-72**
A number of unrelated conditions may result in disseminated intravascular coagulation (DIC). The triggers include direct factors (for example certain tumours) which are capable of initiating coagulation, and indirect factors (for example bacterial endotoxin) which activate coagulation through mediators.

10.15 C D E **Ref: 97, 4073-8**
Haemophilia is an X-linked recessive disorder which usually only affects males clinically. Heterozygous females transmit the disease (as carriers) but may be symptomatically affected when extreme lyonosation results in the preferential expression of the abnormal X chromosome. Thus females may have low levels of Factor VIII, and when these drop to 40-50% of normal activity may be symptomatic when extreme demands are placed on haemostasis (e.g. following major trauma). Although most patients with 25-50% of normal Factor VIII levels do not have clinically significant disease, such low levels can still cause significant and life threatening bleeding following major trauma or surgery.

11. IMMUNOLOGY AND AIDS ANSWERS

11.1 B C D E **Ref: 56, 2308-12**
Malnutrition rather than obesity may cause a depressed immune response. Extremes of life represent periods of increased risk from

Answers : Immunology and AIDS

infection, for example, the elderly are particularly susceptible to pneumococcal pneumonia. Certain infections depress the immune response, classically the lymphotrophic viruses, as in AIDS.

11.2 B C E   **Ref: 56,** 2308-12

Systemic lupus erythematosus is associated with HLA-DR3 but not ankylosing spondylitis which is associated with HLA-B27. Myasthenia gravis is the condition associated with HLA-DR3, not muscular dystrophy.

11.3 D   **Ref: 56,** 2320-5

Hodgkin's disease is linked with varicella zoster, AIDS with *Pneumocystis carinii*, burns with *Pseudomonas aeruginosa* and hyposplenism with pneumococcal sepsis.

11.4 B C   **Ref: 56,** 2320-5

Both *Candida* and *Aspergillus* cause infections in immunocompromised patients but neither are viruses. Herpes viruses (CMV, herpes simplex and varicella zoster) are important causes of viral infections. Echoviruses may cause chronic meningitis in children with hypogammaglobulinaemia.

11.5 A B C D   **Ref: 56,** 2330-3

Non-disposable equipment is best autoclaved following cleaning, even though HIV is quickly inactivated by boiling. Since HIV can survive at ambient temperatures for long periods all surfaces need decontamination. All types of injections are dangerous if contaminated equipment is used. Haemophiliacs are at no risk of being infected by Factor VIII provided that it is heat treated.

11.6 B C   **Ref: 56,** 2330-3

No documented case of transmission of HIV through saliva has been reported. Nine cases of seroconversion following needle-stick injury have been reported, and two cases of possible transmission by breast milk. Household studies have found no evidence of transmission through social contact.

11.7 A B C E   **Ref: 56,** 2334-9

General epidemiological data suggest that the interval between HIV exposure and seroconversion is usually no more than 2 months, and

Answers : Immunology and AIDS

this justifies setting a 3-6 month limit to the follow-up of individuals who have been sexually exposed to HIV infection. Antibody status usually, but not always, indicates the ability of an individual to infect other people; for example, there are several instances of HIV transmission by blood donations from seronegative donors. False-positive antibody tests are not uncommon so all positive results must be cross-checked.

11.8 All False   Ref: 57, 2340-3

The most reliable prognostic marker of the progression of AIDS is the level of CD4 lymphocytes. Falling CD4 levels is a poor prognostic sign, while rising levels is generally interpreted as favourable.

11.9 B D E   Ref: 57, 2340-3

Neither gonorrhoea nor primary syphilis causes generalized lymphadenopathy though secondary syphilis does.

11.10 A E   Ref: 57, 2344-7

Kaposi's sarcoma in patients with AIDS usually develops at several sites simultaneously; the lower limbs are less commonly affected than in classical Kaposi's. There is no evidence that early aggressive treatment improves the prognosis.

11.11 A C D E   Ref: 57, 2344-7

Pneumocystis carinii pneumonia usually has a gradual initial downward course before accelerating with the development of shortness of breath. Sputum seldom contains the causative protozoan unless expectoration is induced by hypertonic saline inhalation.

11.12 A D E   Ref: 57, 2344-7

The mechanism of the neutrophils is still uncertain but the presence of anti-neutrophil antibodies in some patients may suggest an autoimmune basis. Thrombocytopenia is characteristic of AIDS perhaps also due to immunological causes. The anaemia is that of 'chronic disease' so any sudden fall in haemoglobin requires special investigation for other causes.

11.13 A C D E   Ref: 57, 2357-60

Homosexuality appears less common in Africa than elsewhere. Haemophiliacs die young of complications and intravenous drug

Answers : Infection

abuse is uncommon so the most common mode of viral transmission appears to be heterosexual contact. Enteropathic AIDS or 'slim disease' is common in Africa; in some series over 70% of AIDS patients present with chronic diarrhoea. The cause is unknown but may be the protozoan *Cryptosporidium*, *Isospora belli* or *Enterozoa*.

11.14 B D Ref: 57, 2360-3
Up to March 1988 there had been 800 reported cases of fully developed AIDS in children in the US and 20 cases in the UK. Materno-fetal transmission is responsible for 80% of paediatric HIV infections. The ELISA test is not sensitive or specific in young children because of transplacental transfer of maternal antibodies. Live vaccines are not recommended for children with AIDS in the USA and UK, but the WHO recommends that where mortality from natural infections is higher than immunization it should be given, despite the theoretical risks.

11.15 D Ref: 57, 2364-6
The elimination half-life for zidovudine is 1 hour. It penetrates the CSF to provide levels 50-60% of that achieved in plasma which is why it has been used in HIV-related neurological disease, including dementia. Zidovudine is metabolized in the liver which is why one has to be careful with concomitant drug administration e.g. paracetamol, carbemazepine and rifampicin. It may cause nausea and vomiting but these symptoms are usually transient.

12. INFECTION ANSWERS

12.1 A C E Ref: 51, 2077-81
Prior administration of antibiotics may make the bacteraemia of endocarditis difficult to demonstrate microbiologically, but does not make the diagnosis less likely. With the development of non-invasive methods of investigation for PUO, the need for invasive actions has declined.

12.2 A C D Ref: 51, 2082-8
Active, long-lasting immunity can be achieved by using killed, live or toxoid vaccines. Transient, positive immunity is achieved by using antibodies (immunoglobulin) from the plasma of immune individuals.

Answers : Infection

12.3 A B E Ref: 51, 2100-6

Neisseria meningitis is a Gram-negative diplococcus. Occasionally the meningitis is associated with a fulminant septicaemia, septic arthritis and myocarditis.

12.4 A B C D E Ref: 51, 2100-6

Herpes simplex encephalitis is the most common form of sporadic encephalitis in the UK. Post-infectious encephalitis is a rare sequel of measles, chickenpox and other exanthemata and may be a hypersensitivity reaction.

12.5 A C D Ref: 51, 2107-10

Toxoplasmosis is caught by eating infected raw meat or having contact with the faeces of infected birds. The classic triad of features of congenital toxoplasmosis includes hydrocephalus, chorioretinitis and intracranial infection.

12.6 A D E Ref: 52, 2116-21

Bloody diarrhoea is uncommon in yersinia enterocolitis. Diagnosis is commonly by stool or blood culture. Arthritis particularly affects HLA-B27 positive patients. Specific treatment is generally not necessary; tetracycline is effective for protracted bowel symptoms and chloramphenicol for severe systemic disease.

12.7 B C D E Ref: 52, 2127-30

S. typhi depends on human-to-human transfer for its continued existence. The gallbladder is almost always infected, either directly or via the biliary tree and is the commonest cause of chronic infection.

12.8 C D E Ref: 52, 2131-6

Clostridium tetani spores survive for long periods in dust, clothing, hospitals, even the air around wounds and within healed wounds. The neurotoxin is produced by the bacterium, not the spore.

12.9 A B C E Ref: 52, 2136-40

A zoonosis is an infection or infestation shared in nature by man and lower vertebrate animals. First line treatment options include combinations of tetracycline, streptomycin, doxycycline and co-trimoxazole.

Answers : Infection

12.10 A B D Ref: 52, 2141-4
Diphtheria should always be suspected as a cause of croup in a toxic child if cases of diphtheria are occurring in the community. In tropical countries diphtheria may present as a chronic tropical ulcer. Cutaneous diphtheria rarely leads to the classical myocardial and paralytic complications.

12.11 C Ref: 52, 2146-54
Staphylococcus aureus resistance to methicillin and other penicillinase-stable penicillins has produced major epidemics in Australia, the USA and the UK. Ampicillin resistance among *Haemophilus influenzae* has become widespread.

12.12 A C E Ref: 52, 2146-54
Aminoglycosides are effective orally. Renal function, weight, age and sex are important when deciding on appropriate dosage. Antibiotic assays and nomograms are also widely used to make prescribing safer.

12.13 A C D Ref: 52, 2155-63
Tooth pigmentation is linked with tetracycline. Pseudomembranous colitis is linked with clindamycin or lincamycin.

12.14 A B C D E Ref: 53, 2167-71
A haemorrhagic encephalitis of the temporal lobes is, by far, the commonest presentation of herpes encephalitis. The disease has a high mortality though early treatment with acyclovir has produced significant improvements. EEG or CT scan may localize the disease but differentiation from other focal diseases of the brain may require brain biopsy.

12.15 A D E Ref: 53, 2172-5
Epstein-Barr virus is very common in developed countries and particularly in Africa where almost all 5 year olds will have been infected. It is a herpes virus and is closely linked with Burkitt's lymphoma, not leukaemias.

12.16 A C D E Ref: 53, 2177-81
The respiratory complications of measles include pneumonia, pneumomediastinum, bronchiolitis and bronchiectasis but not recurrent pneumothoraces. Severe infection from prolonged and

Answers : Infection

intense exposure to infected siblings in the same household is more likely to cause fatal disease than malnutrition.

12.17 B C D   **Ref: 53, 2187-8**
The first sign of Lyme disease is often the erythematous rash, erythema chronicum migrans, which starts around the tick bite. Sixty per cent of patients develop arthritis and about 8% develop cardiac disorders including pancarditis.

12.18 A B   **Ref: 53, 2189-93**
Immunization should be delayed in a child with gastroenteritis but not other minor infectious diseases. There is no evidence that immunization poses a threat to a pregnant mother or developing fetus but it is usually delayed. When immediate protection is indicated the injected, inactivated vaccine is used.

12.19 A C E   **Ref: 53, 2194-9**
Rabies may be complicated by fluid and electrolyte disturbances including diabetes insipidus (but not mellitus) and inappropriate secretion of antidiuretic hormone. The absence of sensory disturbances is characteristic of rabies.

12.20 A D E   **Ref: 53, 2200-1**
Antibiotics in the early stages of the disease have reduced the mortality for cutaneous anthrax from 20% to about 1%. Gastrointestinal disease is often fatal although there are well-documented cases of recovery.

12.21 A B   **Ref: 54, 2220-5**
In addition to chemoprophylaxis, usually with chloroquine or pyrimethamine, personal protection can be very important. Mosquito nets, mosquito coils, screening of houses, use of insect repellants, spraying of rooms before retiring to bed and clothing covering legs and arms are all useful.

12.22 C E   **Ref: 54, 2247-51**
Dengue fever is transmitted from man to man by mosquitoes. Infection may be asymptomatic, or be associated with a mild fever, or most commonly produces an acute fever with headache, myalgia, arthralgia, rash and leucopenia. Lymphadenopathy is common but

Answers : Infection

liver and spleen are not commonly enlarged. Dengue haemorrhagic fever is much more serious than dengue fever and has a significant mortality.

12.23 D E   Ref: 54, 2251-8

Typhus rickettsia are insensitive to all penicillins and to cotrimoxazole. Clinical response to chloramphenicol and tetracycline is rapid and patients usually improve after 24-48 hours.

12.24 C D   Ref: 55, 2267-9

Humans generally develop hydatid disease from eating infective eggs from the faeces of dogs or wild carnivores. The liver is easily the commonest site for cysts, followed by the lung. The Casoni test is unreliable, with a high level of false positives; serological tests are more reliable.

12.25 A B C D   Ref: 55, 2270-3

The lymphatic vessels of the male genitalia are commonly affected by Bancrofti filariasis producing inflammation of the spermatic cord, epididymitis and orchitis. Hydrocele is the most common sign of chronic bancroftian filariasis. Chyluria usually occurs intermittently, after a heavy meal and may contain mircofilariac even when they are absent in the blood.

12.26 A B E   Ref: 55, 2274-5

An intense eosinophilia (up to 10,000/mm^3) is characteristic of loiasis. Microfilariae are visible in daytime 'fresh' thick blood flims but not nocturnal samples. They can also be seen following fixation and staining with Mayer's haemalum.

12.27 C D   Ref: 55, 2276-9

Onchocerciasis is transmitted by the black fly. There are no important animal reservoirs for onchocerciasis. Onchocerciasis is often called 'river blindness' because the vector lays its eggs attached to submerged rocks and vegetation. No chemoprophylaxis is currently available - the best hope for the future lies in the advent of a macrofilaricide to eliminate the vector.

Answers : Liver Disease

12.28 C D E Ref: 55, 2281-3
Intestinal schistosomiasis is caused by *S. mansoni*. The specific snail host (genus *Biomphalaria*) lives in fresh water. Praziquantel and oxamniquine both have a cure rate of 70-90% and can be given to patients with hepatosplenomegaly.

12.29 A C E Ref: 55, 2291-3
The incubation period for leptospirosis is 2-20 days. Renal failure is observed in 44-67% of hospital cases and is often hypercatabolic with a blood urea: serum creatinine ratio above 30:1. Jaundice occurs in severe forms of leptospirosis but not in most cases.

12.30 B C D E Ref: 55, 2294-7
Some nerves are particularly affected by leprosy, of which the lateral popliteal nerve at the neck of the fibula (causing foot-drop) is one, and the facial nerve (causing lagophthalmos) is another. Testicular atrophy and gynaecomastia are late complications of lepromatous leprosy.

12.31 C Ref: 55, 2298-300
Streptomycin is the drug of choice in the treatment of plague; it may be used in renal failure with caution. Chloramphenicol is valuable for plague meningitis because it penetrates the meninges well. Antibiotic resistance has never been reported and there is no rationale for using multiple antibiotics to treat plague. Buboes usually recede without local therapy.

13. LIVER DISEASE ANSWERS

13.1 D E Ref: 83, 3417-22
A negative urinary urobilinogen is a sensitive and specific test of obstructive jaundice, not much inferior to CT scanning. Almost all bilirubin is metabolized by the liver. Bilirubin is transported bound to albumin.

13.2 D Ref: 83, 3423-30
Oral cholecytography does not work in jaundiced patients and has been largely displaced by ultrasound. CT scanning and ultrasound have replaced nuclear medicine studies in the investigation of liver

Answers : Liver Disease

parenchyma, only 20% of gallstones are radiopaque. Liver secondaries are rarely vascular and so angiography is not successful at visualizing them.

13.3 C   Ref: 83, 3437-44

Hepatitis E is transmitted by the faecal-oral route. It rarely progresses to chronic hepatitis, but has an unusually high mortality rate of 20%. Non-A, non-B hepatitis is hepatitis C.

13.4 A D E   Ref: 83, 3449-52

Hydatid disease is caused by the cestodes, *Ecchinococcus granulosis* or *multilocularis*. Wilson's disease is caused by a genetic enzyme deficiency.

13.5 D   Ref: 83, 3449-52

Hepatic amoebiasis is caused by invasion of the portal circulation by the protozoa *Entamoeba histolytica* during the course of colonic invasion. The protozoa is most commonly found in the tropics, particularly Mexico, Africa and South East Asia and affects 20-50 year old men primarily. Routine needle aspiration of an abscess is not commonly recommended since drug treatment is so successful.

13.6 C E   Ref: 83, 3454-9

Jaundice occurs in both unconjugated and conjugated hyperbilirubinaemia. Other investigations, though, are negative in unconjugated hyperbilirubinaemia, for example urinalysis for bilirubin is negative, liver function tests are normal, the stool is a normal colour and there is no hepatomegaly.

13.7 A D   Ref: 83, 3454-9

Jaundice in childhood can be classified into pre-hepatic, hepatic and cholestatic. The recognised causes of pre-hepatic jaundice include excessive haemolysis characterised by the presence of unconjugated hyperbilirubinaemia; and Gilbert's syndrome, a rare familial, non-haemolytic cause of pre-hepatic jaundice.

13.8 A B D   Ref: 84, 3461-5

Hepatic signs of Wilson's disease usually occur in childhood or adolescence but, very occasionally, they may be present in people aged 25 years and over. Besides methyldopa, other drugs implicated in

Answers : Liver Disease

chronic active hepatitis include nitrofurantoin and oxyphenizatin. Systemic lupus erythematosus does not affect the liver.

13.9　A E　　　　　　　　Ref: 84, 3470-2
Primary biliary cirrhosis is 10 times more common in women than men. It primarily affects people over 65 years and has been only rarely reported in Africa, the Middle East or India. Long-term steroids are contraindicated because of their bone demineralization effect. Osteoporosis is the main bone disorder but treatment with calcium, vitamin D and hydroxyapatite is disappointing.

13.10　A B C E　　　　　　Ref: 84, 3472-83
Vasopressin and nitroglycerin are usually used in combination. Nitroglycerin protects the systemic circulation from the vasoconstrictive effects of vasopressin while maintaining the decrease in splanchnic arteriolar inflow and reduction in portal flow. Somatostatin has virtually no side-effects and seems to have a similar efficacy to vasopressin.

13.11　A C E　　　　　　　Ref: 84, 3472-83
Ascites is the presence of free fluid within the peritoneal cavity - at least 1.5 litres must be present before it can be detected clinically. Decreased plasma colloid pressure due to reduced albumin synthesis is a major factor as is increased hepatic lymph production.

13.12　B E　　　　　　　　Ref: 84, 3484-91
Pigment, rather than cholesterol, stones are associated with bacteria in the bile. Many stones remain asymptomatic; only 30% of patients with stones undergo surgery. Chenodeoxycholic acid is ineffective for pigment stones, heavily calcified stones or stones more than 1.5 cm in diameter.

13.13　A C D　　　　　　　Ref: 84, 3492-5
Hepatocellular carcinoma is linked to hepatitis and not schistosomiasis. Liver biopsy is usually contraindicated because of the risk of precipitating haemorrhage.

13.14　A B D　　　　　　　Ref: 84, 3502-6
Haematological causes of Budd-Chiari syndrome include essential thrombocytosis, polycythaemia rubra vera, paroxysmal nocturnal

haemoglobinuria and early myeloproliferative disorders. Oral contraceptive medication has been associated with Budd-Chiari syndrome but not HRT. Hypernephroma is linked because it can affect the inferior vena cava.

13.15 A B C Ref: 84, 3502-6
Segmental portal hypertension may be the consequence of resection of infarcted gut following inferior or superior mesenteric venous thrombosis. Segmental hypertension may also arise from splenic venous thrombosis and may also be cured by splenectomy. Ascites is a consequence of portal hypertension, not a cause.

14. MULTISYSTEM DISORDERS ANSWERS

14.1 A D Ref: 81, 3328-33
Systemic lupus erythematosus (SLE) is mainly a disease of women in their second and third decade, particularly in South East Asia and the Caribbean where it is more common than rheumatoid arthritis. Concordance between identical twins is 70%. The contraceptive pill often brings on symptoms. Chloroquine is still used for mild disease with cyclophosphamide and azathiprine being reserved for severe illness.

14.2 A B C E Ref: 81, 3335-8
Patients in whom the disease is confined to the skin are described as having CRST syndrome, made up of calcinosis, Raynaud's phenomenon, sclerodactyly and telangiectasia.

14.3 A B C D E Ref: 81, 3338-45
Proteinuria is the most common initial sign of systemic amyloidosis. The macroglossia is part of a diffuse infiltrative process with mass lesions which often mimic other gastrointestinal disorders. Purpura may involve as many as 40% of people with systemic disease.

14.4 B Ref: 81, 3346-8
Polyarteritis nodosa (PAN) affects small and medium sized arteries primarily, but also veins and the vasa nervosa of nerves. Any age group may be affected but the most common is the 30-60-year-old group.

Answers : Neurology

The modern management of PAN includes prednisolone and azathioprine (and cyclophosphamide in severe disease).

15. NEUROLOGY ANSWERS

15.1 A   Ref: 98, 4086-91
Migraine without aura occurs in 75% of patients. Daily headaches are never migrainous. Although migrainous headaches are usually unilateral, they can occasionally be bilateral. Migrainous attacks are probably caused by the release of vasogenic amines from blood vessel walls accompanied by pulsatile distension.

15.2 A C   Ref: 98, 4098-4102
An EEG is not required for the diagnosis of brain stem death in the UK though it is required in many other countries. The EEG is often helpful in diagnosing dementia. For example Creutzfeldt-Jacob disease, Alzheimer's disease and multifocal vascular dementia all show characteristic EEG changes. Most patients with epilepsy show interictal EEG abnormalities but up to 20% may not.

15.3 B C D   Ref: 98, 4098-4102
Although spikes and sharp wave paroxysmal activity are usually associated with epilepsy, it is quite possible to have epilepsy and a normal EEG. Drugs and metabolic disorders severe enough to cause cerebral dysfunction will usually cause EEG abnormalities.

15.4 A E   Ref: 98, 4103-6
The interossei muscles are supplied by the ulnar nerve. Quadriceps is supplied by the femoral nerve while gastrocnemius is supplied by the sciatic nerve.

15.5 A E   Ref: 98, 4106-8
Lumbar puncture is performed by passing a needle into the subarachoid space below the level of the termination of the spinal cord. Needling the aorta is uncommon because the vertebral bodies protect it. Papilloedema is a poor guide to the extent of intracranial pressure, indeed patients can have large intracranial masses without papilloedema being present.

Answers : Neurology

15.6 B D Ref: 98, 4109-13
Multiple sclerosis (MS) has a higher prevalence in temperate than in tropical countries. Hungarian gypsies and the Japanese have an exceptionally low incidence. MS may present with diplopia but it is due to involvement of cranial nerves III, IV or VI, not the optic nerve. MS quite frequently causes sensory disturbance of the limbs.

15.7 C D Ref: 98, 4109-13
Carbamazepine is useful in the treatment of ataxia and some paroxysmal symptoms (including trigeminal neuralgia) but not spasticity. Oxybutynin is used for the treatment of urinary frequency and urgency, and calcium antagonists have a role in the treatment of fatigue.

15.8 C E Ref: 99, 4124-6
Decerebrate and decorticate posturing and epileptic movements all indicate some degree of cerebral function and are incompatible with a diagnosis of brain death. Loss of the light reflex may by due to IIIrd nerve palsy or optic nerve damage complicating head injury, and not due to brain stem death.

15.9 C D E Ref: 99, 4126-30
Hypocalcaemia and hyponatraemia are accepted causes of epileptic fits.

15.10 A C Ref: 99, 4137-42
The side-effects of carbamazepine include diplopia, gait unsteadiness, dizziness, drowsiness and nausea. Hirsutism is a complication of phenytoin. Phenytoin causes connective tissue changes but not weight loss. The side effects of ethosuximide include unsteadiness, headache, drowsiness, ataxia and nausea.

15.11 B E Ref: 99, 4143-7
Hypertension does not appear to be a significant factor in the formation of intracranial aneurysms, but women who smoke are two and a half times more likely to develop aneurysmal subarachnoid haemorrhage than non-smokers. About 90 per cent of aneurysms develop in the anterior communicating, internal carotid and middle cerebral arteries. Multiple aneurysms occur in only about 50 per cent of patients.

Answers : Neurology

15.12 A D Ref: 99, 4143-7
Bleeding from arteriovenous malformations (AVMs) is more commonly intracerebral and subarachnoid and it is for this reason that some experts recommend investigation by arteriography or MRI in all patients under 50 who are not hypertensive and who present with an intracerebral haemorrhage. The risk of death and recurrent haemorrhage are both much lower for AVMs than for aneurysms. AVMs can affect any part of the brain including the cerebellum and brain stem. Patients with AVMs are not automatically treated by surgery, for example those presenting with epilepsy may be treated medically with anticonvulsants.

15.13 A D Ref: 99, 4148-53
Malignant gliomas are the most common intracranial tumours. Meningiomas are seldom seen in childhood or young adulthood; the incidence increases after age 40. Radiotherapy is useful adjunctive treatment for surgically unresectable tumours. Meningiomas have a recurrence rate of 10% at 10 years following resection.

15.14 A B Ref: 99, 4158-67
Stroke is more common in people in lower socio-economic groups, probably because they smoke more and are more likely to suffer from hypertension. About 50% of patients with intracerebral or subarachnoid haemorrhage die within 30 days of their stroke, while in cerebral infarction the mortality is only 10%. Hypertension is the most important risk factor for stroke: in people with a diastolic blood pressure over 100 mm Hg the incidence is about 15 times greater than that of individuals with diastolic pressures below 80 mm Hg.

15.15 B C Ref: 99, 4158-67
The parietal lobe is supplied by the middle cerebral artery and a stroke here causes contralateral upper motor neurone damage. The retina is supplied by the ophthalmic artery and damage to this blood supply causes amaurosis fugax, attitudinal field defects in one eye or complete uniocular blindness.

15.16 D E Ref: 100, 4168-71
Pyridostigmine, 30-120 mg orally, is one of the accepted anticholinesterase treatments for myasthenia gravis. The side-effects are caused by parasympathetic stimulation and include pupillary

Answers : Neurology

constriction, diarrhoea and increased salivation. Propantheline bromide or atropine can be used to control gastrointestinal side-effects.

15.17 A C D   **Ref: 100, 4172-7**
The incidence of Duchenne muscular dystrophy (DMD) is about 18-30 per 10,000 live male births in the developed world. In one third of all patients the disease results from a new mutation; one third of all patients have a family history consistent with X-linked recessive inheritance, and one third are born to carriers. DMD is characterized by the absence of the cytoskeletal protein dystrophin.

15.18 D E   **Ref: 100, 4177-83**
Tremor is the presenting feature in 65% of patients with Parkinson's disease. It tends to affect distal groups of muscles such as those of the hand, forearm and foot. It frequently appears unilaterally before spreading to the other side. The tremor is made worse by nervousness, excitement or fatigue but movement temporarily improves it.

15.19 C D E   **Ref: 100, 4177-83**
Hyperkinesia is characteristic of idiopathic Parkinsonism and is probably the most disabling aspect of the disease. The characteristic drooling of Parkinsonism patients is caused by mechanical factors and not hypersecretion. Dysphagia is common and radiological studies have shown a delay in the initiation of swallowing accompanied by irregular and jerky epiglottic movements.

15.20 A C D   **Ref: 100, 4197-200**
The cause of motor neurone disease (MND) is unknown. The hypothesis about an imbalance between muscle wear and reparative mechanisms is no longer accepted. Nor is the supposed association between excessive physical activity and MND accepted. There is no evidence linking immunological suppression and MND. MND is most common in people over 60. Disease progression is implacable and most patients die within 3-4 years of diagnosis. Respiratory failure is the most common cause of death.

15.21 A B C E   **Ref: 100, 4201-3**
Sarcoidosis may present with isolated facial palsy. Unilateral facial palsy may be an early and predominant feature of Guillain-Barre

syndrome. In Lyme disease there is a rash and sometimes facial induration which may assist diagnosis. In HIV infection accompanying lymphadenopathy may help diagnosis.

15.22 B C D   Ref: 100, 4201-3
Bell's palsy is almost invariably unilateral, indeed the patient may describe his or her face as drawn up on the unaffected side. Sarcoidosis may present as isolated facial palsy. With Lyme disease there may also be a characteristic rash and facial induration. Local lymphadenopathy is often present with HIV infection.

15.23 B D E   Ref: 100, 4201-3
Dry eye caused by denervation of the lacrimal gland is very uncommon, whereas a watering eye is common. The salivary glands are not affected in Bell's palsy. Postauricular pain is common and may precede paralysis by up to two days.

16. NUTRITION ANSWERS

16.1 B C   Ref: 82, 3364-8
Fats provide 9 kcal/g compared with only 4 kcal/g from starchy foods so starchy foods are a useful slimming aid. Overweight people have a higher metabolic rate than people with normal weight, although they often delude themselves otherwise.

16.2 B C D   Ref: 82, 3368-74
Hindmilk is more nutritious than foremilk, containing twice as much fat on average. Vitamin K levels in breast milk are low, which perhaps explains why haemorrhagic disease of the newborn is most common in breast-fed babies. Routine parenteral prophylactic vitamin K 1 mg i.m. or s.c. is effective. An exclusively breast-fed infant will start becoming short of iron at about 6 months.

16.3 B C D E   Ref: 82, 3368-74
Maternal medication seldom constitutes an absolute contraindication to breast feeding; ampicillin presents no particular difficulties. Maternal alcoholism is associated with many difficulties with breast feeding; one serious complication is reduced infantile motor development scores in infants at 1 year. Maternal AIDS may be

dangerous to the infant because transmission of HIV in breast milk seems possible.

16.4 A B C   Ref; 82, 3386-91
Dystrophic changes of hair, skin and nails are characteristic of kwashiorkor rather than marasmus. In children with marasmus age-related weight and height are reduced and despite re-feeding maximal potential is never realized.

16.5 B C E   Ref: 82, 3386-91
Enlarged fatty livers are characteristic of kwashiorkor but not splenomegaly. Diarrhoea rather than constipation is typical. Muscle wasting is usually present though the extent is variable, unlike marasmus where it is usually severe.

16.6 A C   Ref: 82, 3397-401
Thiamine deficiency (or beri-beri) causes, most commonly, a high output biventricular heart failure, preceded by sinus tachycardia, wide pulse pressure and severe sweating. Low output beri-beri has a very poor prognosis. The congestive cardiac failure of selenium deficiency is due to a cardiomyopathy.

16.7 A B C E   Ref: 82, 3405-7
Cobalt salts were used to produce a head on beers in Canada, USA and Belgium. They were banned in 1972 when they were found to cause a cardiac myopathy and some deaths.

17. ONCOLOGY ANSWERS

17.1 A C D   Ref: 92, 3827-9
Far from causing local necrosis some experts advise injecting dexamethasone locally around a site where local infiltration of a toxic drug has taken place. Others, though, feel such action has no proven place.

17.2 A B C D E   Ref: 92, 3834-8
Both squamous and basal cell carcinoma of the skin are responsive to radiotherapy. Radiotherapy is appropriate for locally advanced cervical carcinoma because surgical excision is not possible. Early

Answers : Oncology

anal carcinoma responds well to radiotherapy which has the advantage it does not disturb sphincter function.

17.3 D   **Ref: 92, 3839-41**
Constipation is characteristic of malignant hypercalcaemia rather than diarrhoea. Peripheral sensory loss is not a feature but muscle weakness and lethargy are. Renal failure is a common long term complication of malignant hypercalcaemia but is not due to anuria since polyuria is a recognized symptom. Tetany is due to low serum calcium levels (or alkalosis).

17.4 A C   **Ref: 92, 3839-41**
Symptomatic hypercalcaemia is usually due to carcinoma of the bronchus, breast or kidney or to myeloma or lymphoma. The mechanism is not known; ectopic parathyroid hormone secretion is only very rarely found. Treatment is by diuretics (for example frusemide once rehydration has been completed), calcitonin and diphosphates.

17.5 A B E   **Ref: 92, 3841-3**
Cerebral metastases affect the cerebral hemisphere twice as commonly as the cerebellum. They occur late in the natural history of melanoma.

17.6 A D E   **Ref: 92, 3844-6**
Facial swelling, proptosis and conjunctival oedema occur in superior vena caval obstruction. Neither swelling of the tongue nor nerve deafness is a complication of superior vena caval obstruction.

17.7 B C D E   **Ref: 92, 3844-6**
Neutropenia occurs in some cancers either in isolation or as part of a pancytopenia. It is also seen following chemotherapy or wide-field irradiation.

17.8 A E   **Ref: 92, 3850-4**
Developing countries with traditionally low rates of breast cancer are now experiencing a significant increase in cases. Open biopsy has now been replaced as a diagnostic tool by a combination of fine needle aspiration cytology, mammography and physical examination.

Answers : Oncology

Women with advanced disease are usually treated by radiotherapy rather than chemotherapy.

17.9 B C Ref: 92, 3850-4
Case control studies suggest the risk of breast cancer for women whose menarche occurs before they are 12 years old is almost double that for women who begin menstruating after the age of 13 years. The rapid establishment of regular menstruation increases the risk. High socio-economic class in developed countries is linked with breast cancer, as is early age at birth of first child. Incomplete pregnancies do not seem to provide a protective effect.

17.10 A B D E Ref: 92, 3854-8
Cervical cancer is linked to oral contraceptives, rather than barrier methods of contraception, if the contraceptives have been taken for 10 years or more. Not all of this effect is due to differences in sexual behaviour.

17.11 A C D E Ref: 92, 3854-8
Lymphatic spread is very characteristic of cervical cancer.

17.12 D Ref: 92, 3859-63
Progestogen based oral contraceptives may have a protective effect against endometrial cancer. Endometrial cancer is usually a well-differentiated adenocarcinoma.

17.13 A B C Ref: 92, 3859-63
Ovarian cancer is more common among women with both breast and colonic cancer. Its incidence among Japanese women who move to North America rises to match that of the natives, suggesting an environmental factor (possibly talcum powder applied to the vulva, condoms or diaphragms). Ovarian cancer occurs more commonly among nulliparous and subfertile women than in the general population. Endometrial cancer is the cancer linked with the use of unopposed oestrogen treatment.

17.14 C Ref: 93, 3864-7
Bladder cancer is usually a transitional cell carcinoma. Most tumours at presentation are superficial. Up to 30% of superficial tumours

Answers : Oncology

become invasive, despite adequate treatment. Chemotherapy for metastases improves life expectancy.

17.15 A D   Ref: 93, 3864-7

Prostatic cancer is usually an adenocarcinoma and all types of tumour are found from well differentiated to poorly differentiated. This range of differentiation may even be seen within the same tumour. Prostate-specific antigen is an accurate marker of prostate cancer but not a reliable diagnostic investigation because it can be raised in patients with benign hypertrophy. Prostate cancer responds objectively to hormone therapy in about 40% of cases.

17.16 A D   Ref: 93, 3871-4

Multiple myeloma stimulates osteoclasts to destroy bone. It depresses marrow function and Bence-Jones protein is found in the urine.

17.17 A C D E   Ref: 93, 3871-4

Multiple myeloma commonly presents with bone fractures but they are almost invariably painful - as opposed to metastatic deposits which are often painless.

17.18 B   Ref: 93, 3875-7

The Reed-Sternberg cell is still regarded as the malignant cell in Hodgkin's disease. Biopsy of an enlarged lymph gland is the best diagnostic test. Staging laparotomies are no longer indicated for most patients. Chemotherapy has not improved survival in patients with early disease because toxicity is a major problem for patients receiving this regime. Moreover patients relapsing on radiotherapy alone can be salvaged using chemotherapy.

17.19 B D   Ref: 93, 3882-5

Osteosarcoma is the most common bone tumour. Radiography is an effective diagnostic investigation for most tumours. Surgery in combination with chemotherapy is the modern treatment of choice.

17.20 A C D   Ref: 93, 3888-91

Tuberose sclerosis is associated with an increased risk of brain tumours, Fanconi's anaemia with an increased risk of acute leukaemias and hepatomas, and ataxia telangiectasia with an

Answers : Oral Medicine

increased risk of lymphoreticular, intracranial and gastrointestinal malignancy.

17.21 A D E Ref: 93, 3888-91
Cardiac function is adversely affected by anthracyclines. Pulmonary function is reduced by fibrosis from bleomycin and methotrexate.

18. ORAL MEDICINE ANSWERS

18.1 B C E Ref: 76, 3150-3
Cyclosporin is an important immunosuppressive drug, used for example in preventing graft rejection following transplantation. It may cause gingival swelling. Phenytoin is one of the major treatments for epilepsy but toxic effects are common including hyperplasia of the gums. Nifedipine is a calcium antagonist used for the treatment of angina; it may cause gingival swelling, headache, flushing and palpitations.

18.2 D E Ref: 76, 3154-62
Pigmented mucosal lesions of the mouth are associated with Peutz-Jegher's syndrome but not Plummer-Vinson syndrome. Phenothiazines but not benzodiazepines are linked with oral pigmentation.

18.3 A B E Ref: 76, 3154-62
Several studies have shown an association between high alcohol consumption and oral cancer; for example in Brittany between the pot-stilled spirit calvados and cancer of the mouth. Iron deficiency, as in the Plummer-Vinson syndrome, but not folate deficiency, predisposes to oral cancer. Cigar smoking is associated with leukoplakia of the floor of the mouth in women.

18.4 B D E Ref: 76, 3167-9
Tricyclic but not monoamine oxidase inhibitor antidepressants cause a dry mouth, as do bronchodilators but not bronchoconstrictors.

Answers : Poisoning

19. POISONING ANSWERS

19.1 A B D Ref: 61, 2496-8
Girls are more likely to attempt suicide (peak incidence 14-16 years of age), but boys are more likely to succeed. The incidence of intentional self-poisoning in the over 60 year age group is higher (20%) than the average (13%) for the whole population. Causes include bereavement (self-poisoning occurs on anniversaries), loneliness, failing health and loss of independence.

19.2 A D Ref: 61, 2508-12
Protamine is an appropriate antidote for heparin overdosage. Flumazenil is an appropriate antidote for benzodiazepines and desferrioxamine mesylate for lead. Penicillamine is useful for acute and chronic arsenic poisoning and for mercury poisoning.

19.3 A D Ref: 61, 2513-6
Toxins which are poorly absorbed by activated charcoal include acids and alkalis, ethanol, ethylene glycol, iron, lithium and methanol.

19.4 C D E Ref: 61, 2516-21
Severe salicylate intoxication (plasma concentrations 800-1000 mg/litre) may cause hypotension and cardiac arrest. Deafness, bradycardia, tinnitus and sweating are recognized complications of moderate intoxication (500-800 mg/litre).

19.5 A D E Ref: 61, 2522-5
In theophylline poisoning hypotension is due to reduced peripheral resistance not reduced cardiac output. Hyperventilation occurs following stimulation of respiratory centres. Diarrhoea, abdominal cramps and pain and gastrointestinal haemorrhage are all local gastrointestinal effects.

19.6 A B C E Ref: 61, 2526-9
Disc batteries more than 20 mm in diameter may become stuck in the oesophagus causing obstruction, so chest radiographs are always indicated. Petroleum distillates give cause for concern because they may be aspirated into the respiratory tract where they spread evenly because of their low surface tension. The most common respiratory complication of petroleum distillate poisoning is haemorrhagic

Answers : Psychiatry

pneumonitis which is difficult to treat and occasionally fatal. Ingestion of strong acids should be treated by milk (or similar fluid) to dilute and neutralize the acid followed by supportive measures as necessary.

19.7 D E   Ref: 61, 2530-4

Chronic lithium poisoning is more common than acute poisoning. Clinical features tend to relate closely to plasma levels except in acute poisoning. Diarrhoea, hypokalaemia and hypotension are possible complications of lithium poisoning.

20. PSYCHIATRY ANSWERS

20.1 B C E   Ref: 94, 3904-8

Most studies indicate that a working class background predisposes to major depression. Unemployment, rather than continuous employment, is a major factor in the aetiology of depression.

20.2 A C E   Ref: 94, 3904-8

Most patients with psychotic as well as depressive symptoms need an antipsychotic drug or ECT in addition to antidepressive treatment to achieve recovery. ECT is often helpful for patients with schizophrenic symptoms. ECT causes short-term memory loss but this is almost invariably transient.

20.3 A E   Ref: 94, 3917-22

A known precipitating cause and acute onset of illness in schizophrenia are both good prognostic indicators. Prominent affective symptoms and catatonic symptoms are also good indicators.

20.4 A B C   Ref: 94, 3917-22

The incidence of schizophrenia appears similar worldwide although the prognosis appears better in developing countries such as India or parts of Africa. Schizophrenia certainly has some genetic links but is not an autosomal dominant illness. Concordance rates in twins reared both together and apart show rates of 50-60% compared with about 12% for siblings. Recent research has suggested a genetic locus on chromosome 5 in some cases of familial schizophrenia but this work has yet to be corroborated.

Answers : Psychiatry

20.5 D E   **Ref: 94, 3932-6**
Monitoring of lithium levels is necessary because there is wide individual variation in renal lithium clearance, and the dose required for optimal anti-manic effect is only slightly less than that resulting in toxicity. Some drugs, for example diuretics and non-steroidal anti-inflammatory drugs may affect plasma levels. The latter group of drugs, for example, may raise plasma lithium levels.

20.6 C D E   **Ref: 94, 3932-6**
Reduced appetite and difficulty sleeping are recognized side-effects of 5-HT uptake inhibitors.

20.7 C E   **Ref: 94, 3932-6**
Lithium causes a fine rather than coarse tremor. It causes hyperglycaemia and leucocytosis (rather than neutropenia).

20.8 A C E   **Ref: 94, 3932-6**
Blurred vision, constipation and tachycardia are anticholinergic effects of tricyclic antidepressants. Drowsiness is an α_1-adrenoceptor blockade effect. Weight gain is both a histamine H_1-receptor blockade effect and a $5H_2$ receptor effect.

20.9 A B   **Ref: 95, 3950-2**
Surprisingly, women who have had obstetric complications do not seem to suffer more from postnatal depression. Suicide attempts by women shortly after birth are very rare. Antidepressant drugs are secreted only in small amounts into breast milk so treatment by them using moderate dosages is safe.

20.10 A C   **Ref: 95, 3950-2**
Puerperal psychosis commonly begins in the first week postpartum following a 'lucid interval' of several days. The early signs are non-specific and include mood changes, irritability and sleeplessness. The modern management of puerperal psychosis includes trying to keep mother and child together in specialized mother and baby units. Recovery usually takes 2-3 months but the risk of recurrence after a subsequent delivery is about 35%.

20.11 A B D   **Ref: 95, 3953-8**

The greater the number of stressful life events (such as death, sickness, redundancy, moving home) the more likely it becomes for child abuse to occur. Such stressors are more likely to cause fathers to abuse than mothers. And stressors alone are not sufficient to lead to violence; they must be combined with factors such as models of family violence. Time spent interacting closely with family members may lead to irritation and abusive acts towards those members, reinforcing the cycle of violence.

20.12 C E   **Ref: 95, 3963-7**

Solvent abuse causes a disinhibited, excited state which usually disappears within a few minutes. Death from toxic effects on the brain, heart, lungs and liver have been reported but not from renal failure.

20.13 D E   **Ref: 95, 3972-4**

Anorexia nervosa occurs in about 0.5-1% of adolescent and young adult women, and clinically significant bulimia nervosa is seen in 2% of women. Many bulimics are of normal weight, unlike anorexics who usually appear emaciated. Some patients with bulimia will respond to antidepressant medication, preferably those with minimum antihistamine and anticholinergic properties. The long term effect of these drugs in bulimia, however, is not known.

20.14 B D   **Ref: 95, 3975-7**

People with Down's syndrome are prone to hypothyroidism - as many as 35% have circulating thyroid antibodies. Clinical recognition is difficult because they are shorter than average, slower, less active and less alert and occasionally have a hoarse voice. Postmortem studies of people with Down's syndrome have confirmed that a high proportion have pathological changes indistinguishable from Alzheimer's disease.

21. RENAL DISORDERS ANSWERS

21.1 B C D E   **Ref: 85, 3516-21**

Reduced muscle mass (which may occur in the elderly, in the young and in patients with wasting disease) reduces measured plasma creatinine level. Severe renal failure also causes a reduced muscle

Answers : Renal Disorders

mass, increased tubular secretion and intestinal destruction of creatinine.

21.2 A C E   Ref: 85, 3516-21
Glomerular filtration rate may be estimated from plasma urea measurements. However urea production is rapidly affected by protein intake and fluctuates more widely during the day than creatinine. Any liver damage (including hepatitis) will reduce urea production. Doxycycline (in contrast to tetracycline) does not raise plasma urea.

21.3 A C E   Ref: 85, 3522-32
Fluid deprivation is advocated to improve the visibility of the renal outlines during the pyelogram but has become less necessary with the use of higher doses of contrast media. Dehydration should be avoided in the very young and old, and patients with renal impairment (e.g. diabetes or myelomatosis).

21.4 A   Ref: 85, 3522-32
Renal ultrasonography delineates renal parenchyma well and is useful for perirenal collections and non-opaque stones. Small caliceal lesions, however, may be difficult to detect because of masking from sinus fat around the pelvicalyceal system.

21.5 A D   Ref: 85, 3533-5
All adults with nephrotic syndrome should be biopsied. There is little information to be gained from biopsying patients with cystic kidney disease or nephrolithiasis. Biopsy is useful in determining the cause and prognosis of patients with end-stage renal failure.

21.6 A B   Ref: 85, 3533-5
The presence of the nephrotic syndrome is one of the major indications for biopsy. A shrunken kidney is difficult to locate and biopsy and may be a reason for avoiding the procedure. Intravenous diazepam makes biopsy considerably less worrying and painful and may induce amnesia for the event.

21.7 B C E   Ref: 85, 3535-8
During pregnancy both the glomerular filtration rate and plasma flow increase by approximately 40-50% starting from the fourth week of

161

gestation and reaching a peak at about 16 weeks. Bacteriuria accompanies pregnancy in 5-10% of women; recently it was found that up to 40% of untreated patients will develop acute pyelonephritis. So bacteriuria merits prompt treatment.

21.8 A C D E   Ref: 85, 3535-8
Pre-eclampsia seldom recurs after the first pregnancy unless it is a manifestation of latent essential hypertension or occurs as a complication of renal disease when it will recur in all subsequent pregnancies. Pre-eclampsia is treated by bed-rest, antihypertensive drugs (preferably methyldopa) and induction if appropriate.

21.9 A B D E   Ref: 86, 3548-52
Glomerulonephritis is equally common in lepromatous and non-lepromatous leprosy. Bancoftian filariasis, common in Africa and South East Asia, causes mesangial or diffuse proliferative glomerulonephritis. Quartan malarial nephropathy primarily affects children and young adults; it is thought to be mediated by an immune complex. Antimalarial treatment does not alter the course of renal disease, but prednisolone or cyclophosphamide may induce partial or complete remission. In loa-loa infection membranous, mesangio-capillary and chronic sclerosing glomerulonephritis have been reported.

21.10 A D   Ref: 86, 3553-62
Glomerular dysfunction commonly causes hypercoagulability perhaps due to the increased production of certain plasma constituents (e.g. clotting factors) combined with the increased urinary loss of others (e.g. antithrombin III). Low circulating levels of 25-hydroxycalciferol, which is lost with its binding protein in the urine, and of 1,25-dihydroxycholecalciferol results in decreased bone mobilization and gut absorption of calcium. This causes hypocalcaemia. Hypercholesterolaemia occurs in patients with nephrotic syndrome, primarily due to a rise in low density lipoprotein cholesterol. More severe protein loss may cause hypertriglyceridaemia and a concomitant increase in very low density lipoproteins.

21.11 B D   Ref: 86, 3565-8
Muscle cramps are linked to frusemide. Cutaneous flushing, an increase in headaches and fluid retention are complications of calcium

Answers : Renal Disorders

agonists. Hirsutism is a complication of the powerful vasodilator minoxidil.

21.12 C D E Ref: 86, 3569-75
Cataracts and hyperglycaemia are side-effects of corticosteroids. Generally, complications of cyclosporin are dose-dependent.

21.13 A D E Ref: 86, 3569-75
Infective complications of continuous ambulatory peritoneal dialysis (CAPD) may be the most serious which face the patient. Coagulase-negative staphylococci such as *Staphylococcus epidermis* are the most common organisms. Others include *Klebsiella* spp., *Enterobacter* spp. and *Escherichia coli*. Another CAPD complication is exacerbation of pre-existing hyperlipidaemia in some patients following the use of large volumes of high osmolar fluid to improve ultrafiltration.

21.14 C D E Ref: 86, 3578-85
Sulphonamides can cause obstructive uropathy due to crystal obstruction; or they can cause a renal vasculitis. They do not cause an acute tubular necrosis. Tetracyclines cause acute renal failure by reason of hypercatabolism.

21.15 A C Ref: 86, 3585-8
90% of children with nocturnal enuresis are dry during the day. By the age of 10 years, 7% of children wet their beds at least once a week. Urodynamic studies do not often help diagnose the cause of nocturnal enuresis. It is not known how the tricyclic anti-depressants (e.g. imipramine) achieve temporary dryness, but it does not seem to be related to their anticholinergic or antidepressant effect or their local anaesthetic effect on the bladder.

21.16 C D Ref: 87, 3596-600
Cystinosis and Hartnup's syndrome are autosomal recessive conditions. Familial hypophosphataemia is X-linked.

21.17 A C E Ref: 87, 3601-3
Fanconi's syndrome is characterized by aminoaciduria, excess urinary phosphate, glycosuria, tubular acidosis and phosphaturia. The

Answers : Renal Disorders

syndrome includes cystinosis, idiopathic 'adult' Fanconi's syndrome and secondary Fanconi's syndrome.

21.18 All False Ref: 87, 3604-10
Urinary tract infection (UTI) affects approximately 25-35% of all women some time in their lives. The incidence has not fallen since the introduction of antibiotics. Although UTI affects women more than men, this is not true in people over 65 years of age. UTI is usually a single organism infection of which *Escherichia coli* is the most common organism. *Pseudomonas* spp. particularly infects the urinary tract following instrumentation.

21.19 A B C D Ref: 87, 3610-17
Although most children come to no harm from urinary tract infection (UTI) the fundamental objective is to identify those at risk of developing permanent renal damage. Diagnosis of UTI usually requires pure urinary culture of 10^3/ml. Single antibiotics are usually preferred for treatment, for example trimethoprim or cefadroxil.

21.20 B C E Ref: 87, 3625-31
Renal tubular acidosis tends to cause calcium stones, as does medullary sponge kidney where small stones collect within the characteristic ballooning (ectasia) of the final ductules which open into the calceal system.

21.21 C D E Ref: 87, 3632-4
Silastic catheters are favoured for long-term drainage because they are less irritant than silicone coated ones. Catheter sizes are classified according to the Charriere or French system whereby the size is the external diameter in millimetres multiplied by three.

21.22 C E Ref: 87, 3635-6
Renal cell carcinoma is uncommon in children, but is the most common adult renal tumour. It arises from the proximal convoluted tubule and is best treated by surgery alone including surgery of one or two metastases, following which the prognosis may still be good. Hypercalcaemia due to parathyroid hormone production is a recognized presentation finding.

Answers : Respiratory Disorders

22. RESPIRATORY DISORDERS ANSWERS

22.1 A D E Ref: 88, 3640-3
The likelihood of developing lung cancer is influenced by genetic factors. There is considerable current interest in the expression of oncogenes in lung cancer cell lines. There is a strong association between infant respiratory diseases and parental smoking, but this association has almost disappeared by adolescence.

22.2 A C E Ref: 88, 3650-61
Allergic aspergillosis characteristically causes bronchial wall thickening but not septal lines. Hydatid disease causes cysts which appear as intracavity bodies.

22.3 A B C E Ref: 88, 3650-61
Nitrofurantoin causes basal interstitial opacities but not pleural effusion.

22.4 A E Ref: 88, 3661-8
In health the millions of small airways (under 3 mm in size) contribute very little to airway resistance; most is contributed by the large airways. Reducing gas density increases its flow along a tube. An increase in compliance usually reduces flow because elastic recoil of the lung fails. By contrast, people with reduced compliance usually maintain flow well.

22.5 C D E Ref: 88, 3661-8
Carbon monoxide gas transfer (TLCO) is raised by polycythaemia because it raises the level of available haemoglobin in the capillaries. Similarly, alveolar haemorrhage increases the amount of haemoglobin available to carbon monoxide within the alveoli.

22.6 B D Ref: 88, 3669-72
A myocardial infarction within the last six months is usually accepted as the cut-off point for bronchoalveolar lavage (BAL). BAL is certainly more hazardous in the presence of asthma but it is not a contraindication. Quite the contrary, it may be a useful diagnostic tool provided bronchodilator therapy has been administered prior to lavage.

Answers : Respiratory Disorders

22.7   A B E Ref: 88, 3673-5
Paediatric bronchoscopes are useful for viewing lesions distal to sub-segmental level but they cannot be used for biopsy. About 70% of lung cancers are visible at bronchoscopy.

22.8   B E Ref: 88, 3679-82
Acute pulmonary oedema is a complication of hydrochlorothiazide, alveolitis of azathioprine and lupus syndrome of hydralazine.

22.9   C Ref: 89, 3684-6
Acute epiglottitis (EP) is usually caused by *Haemophilus influenzae* type B. It affects children aged 2-3 years most commonly. Clinical examination of the neck and lateral radiograph of the neck are both dangerous manoeuvres which can precipitate complete airway obstruction. Direct laryngoscopy is the examination of preference, under halothane and oxygen in theatre by an experienced anaesthetist, with an airway established. EP rarely recurs.

22.10 A B C E Ref: 89, 3687-8
Chest radiographs in both inspiration and expiration are useful in the investigation of a suspected foreign body inhalation. Expiratory films can show the affected lung failing to change volume in expiration as compared with the unaffected lung.

22.11 B D Ref: 89, 3689-94
Pulmonary cystic fibrosis is not present at birth: it is commonly precipitated by a viral infection followed by a bacterial infection. This infection leads to hypertrophy and dilatation of mucus glands which causes obstruction and secondary infection and the initiation of the vicious circle which eventually leads to progressive lung damage. The primary physiological abnormality is small airway obstruction. The residual volume increases rapidly.

22.12 D Ref: 89, 3703-7
Skin allergy tests are generally uninformative and should not be ordered routinely. Chest radiographs are only indicated for acute episodes if complications are suspected. Pulmonary function tests become reliable in children aged 7-8 years and over. IgE and radio-allergosorbent tests are not indicated in the management of childhood asthma.

Answers : Respiratory Disorders

22.13 A D E Ref: 89, 3712-14
Car spray-painting is linked with isocyanates and metal plating with nickel.

22.14 A B C E Ref: 89, 3718-21
After standardization for smoking, men are still more at risk than women of chronic obstructive airways disease. Homozygous serum-protease inhibitor deficiency is the strongest single risk factor but not intermediate deficiency which is unimportant.

22.15 B D E Ref: 89, 3722-6
Theophylline is eliminated primarily (about 90%) by hepatic metabolism. Blood levels may be needed to establish an appropriate dosage because of wide inter-individual variation in the rate of metabolism; plasma half-lives in normal individuals vary from six to twelve hours.

22.16 A B C D E Ref: 90, 3732-9
Pneumococcal pneumonia is the most common community acquired infection and probably accounts for most cases where no cause is identified, usually because of prior antibiotic therapy. The most common atypical organism is *Mycoplasma pneumoniae*. Pneumonia ranks third behind urinary tract infections and wound infections in frequency of hospital acquired infections.

22.17 B D E Ref: 90, 3739-42
There is generally a latent period of 15-40 years between exposure to asbestos and disease. Following diagnosis, symptomatic treatment is all that can usefully be offered.

22.18 A Ref: 90, 3743-5
Tuberculosis is the most common opportunistic infection in African patients with AIDS; by contrast to Europe where *Pneumocystis carinii* is the likeliest diagnosis. Bilateral perihilar shadowing is the characteristic finding on radiography. Approximately 10% of patients with *P. carinii* have a normal chest radiograph. Antibodies to *P. carinii* are not helpful in diagnosis. Bronchoalveolar lavage, using the fibreoptic bronchoscope, diagnoses *P. carinii* pneumonia in over 90% of cases.

Answers : Respiratory Disorders

22.19 C D E   Ref: 90, 3746-52

Isoniazid, rather than rifampicin, potentiates anticonvulsants. Thiacetazone may cause conjunctivitis.

22.20 D E   Ref: 90, 3753-6

Pulmonary sarcoidosis often remits spontaneously. It is most common between the ages of 20-30.

22.21 D   Ref: 90, 3757-61

About 50% of patients with cryptogenic fibrosing alveolitis (CFA) die within 5 years. CFA commonly presents between 50 and 60 years of age. Finger clubbing occurs in 66-85% of patients. No known initiating stimulus is recognized for CFA so it cannot be classified as an occupational disease.

22.22 C D   Ref: 90, 3762-4

Progressive massive fibrosis is characterized by radiological opacities greater than 10 mm in diameter which may subsequently grow to occupy as much as a third of the lung. Upper lobes are affected first.

22.23 A B C   Ref: 90, 3762-4

Studies in the UK and Germany have shown that the risk of developing coalworker's pneumonia (CP) is related to the dose of coal inhaled. CP is not associated with either an increased risk of tuberculosis or lung cancer.

22.24 D   Ref: 91, 3776-80

Pulmonary oedema, not lobar pneumonia, is characteristic of adult respiratory distress syndrome (ARDS). The absence of haemodynamic factors, such as left ventricular failure, is necessary to diagnose ARDS. Platelets usually fall, but fibrinogen degradation products increase. Lung compliance falls causing an increase in the work of breathing and a fall in functional residual capacity.

22.25 A C D   Ref: 91, 3785-8

Mechanical ventilation is used for the therapeutic manipulation of $PaCO_2$ levels to control cerebral blood flow, particularly following head injury.

Answers : Rheumatology

22.26 A B E Ref: 91, 3789-93
Adenocarcinoma occurs amongst non-smokers and squamous cell carcinoma among smokers. No genetic association has been clearly established for lung cancer.

22.27 B D E Ref: 91, 3805-7
Most mediastinal asymptomatic masses are benign. Fine needle aspiration is not recommended for biopsy of mediastinal masses.

22.28 B C D Ref: 91, 3808-14
Neutrophils predominate in pleural fluid when there is an acute infection. Cholesterol crystals are found in the presence of some chronic effusions (e.g. rheumatoid disease).

22.29 A E Ref: 91, 3814-16
Patients with significant coronary disease are not suitable for lung transplantation. Patients requiring assisted ventilation have a very poor prognosis following transplantation and are therefore not suitable. Lung transplantation cannot be offered on an emergency basis.

22.30 A B C D E Ref: 91, 3817-20
A necrotizing inflammatory process may weaken the wall of a bronchus leading to dilatation and bronchiectasis. This is seen in tuberculosis and histoplasmosis. In measles and pertussis pneumonia, exposive coughing may contribute to dilatation of the bronchial wall, weakened by the inflammatory process. In allergic aspergillosis antigen-antibody complexes are found in the bronchial wall which may lead to an inflammatory reaction and wall destruction.

23. RHEUMATOLOGY ANSWERS

23.1 A C D Ref: 74, 3057-60
Cyst formation and trabecular collapse are characteristic of osteoarthritis, often accompanied by subchondral sclerosis and osteophyte formation. Synovial proliferation and turbid, inflammatory synovial fluid are characteristic of rheumatoid arthritis.

Answers : Rheumatology

23.2 B C D Ref: 74, 3060-6
Rheumatoid factors (RFs) may be epiphenomena of rheumatoid disease or may be involved in some way with the pathogenesis but certainly do not cause the disease. RFs are often found in patients with non-arthritic conditions, especially those with chronic inflation and infection. RFs are produced locally in joints and may form complexes with the ability to start the complement cascade. Treatment has no effect upon the presence of RFs in the bloodstream.

23.3 D E Ref: 74, 3067-72
Depression is a well-recognized feature of rheumatoid arthritis (RA) and must be sought in every patient. Generalized lymphadenopathy affects about 50% of patients with active RA. Occasionally one node is so disproportionately large that it must be biopsied to exclude lymphoma.

23.4 A B C Ref: 74, 3073-8
Ankylosing spondylitis was once considered an uncommon disease but it is now known it has a similar prevalence to rheumatoid arthritis. It was also thought to affect males predominantly but recent studies have shown a comparable distribution between the sexes. Elevation of the ESR occurs in 50% of patients but may be normal despite severe disease.

23.5 A C E Ref: 74, 3073-8
Dysentery caused by *Shigella*, *Salmonella*, *Yersinia* and *Campylobacter* is commonly linked with Reiter's syndrome (RS). Sex distribution is difficult to define because urethritis in women is often clinically inapparent; however males do not outnumber females by ten to one and the post-dysenteric RS has an equal sex distribution. RS is rarely self-limiting - 80% of patients have evidence of disease activity on re-examination after five years and many have major disability.

23.6 B C E Ref: 74, 3079-80
Pseudogout is acute pyrophosphate arthropathy caused by the shedding into the joint of preformed calcium pyrophosphate dihydrate crystals from deposits mainly in fibrocartilage. Systemic features such as fever and confusion are common. Pseudogout resolves spontaneously within 1-3 weeks in most cases.

Answers : Rheumatology

23.7 C D   Ref: 74, 3080-4

Children tolerate non-aspirin non-steroidal anti-inflammatory drugs (NSAIDs) better than adults, as a general rule. Many doctors use high-dose corticosteroids in the treatment of systemic disease, for example initial daily dosages of 30-60 mg/day have been used. Other doctors, though, regard them as valuable only once non-aspirin NSAIDs have failed. Methotrexate appears to have a safer profile than other anti-metabolites and is probably the drug of choice if an anti-metabolite is indicated.

23.8 D E   Ref: 74, 3095-8

The already low incidence of polymyositis and dermatomyositis decreases with age. The importance of these two conditions in elderly people is their putative association with malignancy. In recent years the validity of this association has been questioned but nevertheless the usual screening tests are probably indicated. Elderly onset of scleroderma and systemic lupus erythematosus is unusual.

23.9 B C E   Ref: 75, 3100-4

The reason magnetic resonance imaging (MRI) is becoming so important to rheumatologists is that it successfully differentiates between soft tissues. Pacemakers and artery clips are contraindications to MRI.

23.10 D   Ref: 75, 3105-9

Hyperkalaemia is linked with non-steroidal anti-inflammatory drugs (NSAIDs). Red cell aplasia and haemolytic anaemia are linked with NSAIDs rather than polycythaemia.

23.11 A D E   Ref: 75, 3110-6

Azathioprine is linked with non-Hodgkin's lymphoma and antimalarials with eye toxicity.

23.12 B E   Ref: 75, 3126-31

Standard radiography is not a reliable technique for diagnosing stress fractures. More effective are ultrasound and bone scintography. The lower limb, pelvis, metatarsal, lower tibia, fibula and femoral neck are the most common sites for stress fractures. Spot tenderness is a usual though not invariable sign of stress fracture.

23.13 A B E Ref: 75, 3132-5

The annual incidence of gout in the UK is about 0.3/1000 population; elsewhere in Western Europe the prevalence is higher rising to 15/1000 among French men aged 33-44 years. The reason for the male predominance is not known. Two types of people are particularly affected: obese, male heavy drinkers of alcohol and elderly patients taking thiazide diuretics.

23.14 A Ref: 75, 3136-40

Hypertrophic pulmonary osteoarthropathy is associated with swelling, oedema and effusions of the knees, ankles and wrists. Amyloid causes a rheumatoid-like arthritis commonly affecting hands, shoulders and knees. Acromegaly affects knees, hips and shoulders symmetrically and may proceed to a disabling osteoarthritis. Behçet's syndrome causes a polyarteritis resembling a spondyloarthropathy.

24. SEXUALLY TRANSMITTED DISEASES ANSWERS

24.1 D Ref: 72, 2981-2

Anaerobic vaginosis (AV) is a multibacterial infection in which *Gardnerella vaginalis* and *Bacteroides* play an important role. The vaginal pH rises in AV to about 5.5 and this rise may contribute to the development of the condition. AV is not a sexually transmitted disease but it occurs only in sexually active women for reasons that are not fully understood. Perhaps the rise in pH caused by the introduction of seminal fluid may be an important factor. AV is best treated by metronidazole.

24.2 C D E Ref: 72, 2983-5

Chlamydia trachomatis causes conjunctivitis, otitis media and afebrile pneumonia in neonates. Epididymitis develops in 1-2% of men with untreated non-specific urethritis and is usually caused by *Chlamydia trachomatis*.

24.3 B E Ref: 72, 2988-92

The incubation period for genital warts is up to nine months, and recurrence is common. Most warts are caused by various genotypes of the human papilloma virus. The incidence of warts in women has risen faster than in men for reasons that are not fully understood; it

Answers : Sexually Transmitted Diseases

may be associated with the sub-clinical nature of cervical infection in women.

24.4 C   Ref: 72, 2996-9

Meningovascular syphilis is a feature of quaternary syphilis and may present as a low-grade meningitis with accompanying cranial nerve lesions. Aortitis and tabes dorsalis are also features of quaternary not tertiary syphilis. Osteoporosis is not a complication of tertiary syphilis but osteoperiostitis is, notably of the tibia.

24.5 A B D E   Ref: 72, 3003-6

Early age of first sexual intercourse, age under 25, multiple sexual partners or recent change of sexual partner are all risk factors for PID. Similarly recent pregnancy or any recent gynaecological procedure are associated with PID.

24.6 B E   Ref: 72, 3014-17

Lymphogranuloma venereum is caused by *Chlamydia trachomatis* and has an incubation period of 7-28 days. The primary stage is characterized by a genital vesicle or papule which becomes an ulcer. The secondary stage is marked by lymphadenitis. Erythromycin is safe and effective for pregnant women at a dose of 500 mg qds for 14 days.

24.7 B C D E   Ref: 72, 3014-17

Granuloma inguinale is characterized by the absence of inguinal lymph gland enlargement, unless there is secondary infection. Sometimes a subcutaneous granuloma in the inguinal region (pseudobulo) may be mistaken for inguinal lymphadenopathy.

24.8 A C   Ref: 73, 3020-4

Genital herpes usually starts within 1 week of exposure. Recurrent attacks are usually unrelated to sexual intercourse, the ulcers being small in number and confined to one site. Inguinal lymphadenopathy and general malaise are frequently present.

24.9 A C   Ref: 73, 3034-5

The signs of neonatal gonococcal infection (NGI) usually first appear 1-12 days following delivery. Disseminated disease occurs in only a few babies with NGI. Neural deafness is not a complication of NGI.

Answers : Sexually Transmitted Diseases

24.10 D E　　　　　　　　**Ref: 73,** 3043-5

The myopathy of osteomalacia is generally proximal. Serum alkaline phosphatase levels are usually (but not invariably) raised in osteomalacia, except for the rare congenital hypophosphataemia. The specific radiological features of osteomalacia include pseudofractures, known as Looser's zones or Milkman fractures.

24.11 B C D E　　　　　　**Ref: 73,** 3043-5

Familial hypophosphataemic rickets is a sex-linked dominant disorder. It responds poorly to both 1,25 dihydroxy vitamin D as well as vitamin D, suggesting impaired vitamin D metabolism is not responsible.

24.12 B C E　　　　　　　**Ref: 73,** 3049-50

Alkaline phosphatase is produced by osteoblasts and probably plays an essential role in the calcification of unmineralized osteoid. Serum levels therefore reflect the lyosomal enzyme, acid phosphatase.

24.13 B E　　　　　　　　**Ref: 73,** 3049-50

Parathyroid hormone (PTH) is secreted in response to hypocalcaemia; there is no releasing factor. PTH increases skeletal calcium turnover and may increase serum calcium. PTH only acts indirectly on the small intestine to increase calcium absorption. It stimulates renal 1-hydroxylase to convert 25-hydroxycholecalciferol to 1,25 hydroxycholecalciferol, the active metabolite of vitamin D.

INDEX

5-HT uptake inhibitors 79
ACE inhibitors 5
Acne vulgaris 23
Acromegaly 26
Active immunity 48
Acute tubular necrosis 85
Addison's disease 27
Adenocarcinoma, gastric 31
Adult respiratory distress
    syndrome 18, 94
AIDS, haematological
    abnormalities 46
    in Africa 47
    in children 47
    Kaposi's sarcoma 46
    prognostic markers 45
    zidovudine treatment 47
Alcohol, consumption 1
    dependence syndrome 1
    withdrawal 2
Aminoglycosides 50
Amyloidosis, systemic 60
Anaemia, aplastic 41
Anaerobic vaginosis 100
Aneurysms, left ventricular 6
    intracranial 63
Angiography, coronary 7
Angioplasty 7
    femoral 9
Ankylosing spondylitis 96
Antagonists 13
Antedepressants, tricyclic 79
Antenatal investigations 38
Anthrax 52
Antibiotics and side effects 51
Antidiuresis, inappropriate 27
Antithrombotic drugs 14
Aorta, coarctation 10
Aortic regurgitation 11
    stenosis, congenital 11
    valvotomy 11
Aplastic anaemia 41

Appendicitis, acute 33
Arteries 64
Arteriovenous malformations 63
Arthritis in children 97
Asbestosis 92
Ascites, hepatic 58
Asthma, in children 91
    occupational 91
Autonomic function tests 24

Barium meal, double contrast 31
Basal cell carcinoma 22
Bell's palsy 66
Biliary tract 56
Biopsy, percutaneous renal 83
Bladder cancer 72
Blood pressure 8, 9
Bone 102
    tumours 73
Bowel disease, ischaemic 36
Bowen's disease 23
Bradycradia 4
Brain death, diagnosis 62
Breast cancer 70, 71
Breast-feeding 15, 67
    contraindications 67
Bronchiectasis 95
Bronchoalveolar lavage, elective 89
Bronchoscopy, fibreoptic 89
Brucellosis 50
Budd-Chiari syndrome 59
Bulimia nervosa 81

Calcium-channel blockers 14
Cancer, bladder 72
    breast 70, 71
    cervical 71
    colorectal 35
    endometrial 71
    lung 94
    oral 75
    ovarian 72
    pancreatic 32

Index

prostatic 72
Cannabis 2
Carbon monoxide gas transfer 89
Carcinoma, basal cell 22
  hepatocellular 59
  papillary thyroid 26
  renal cell 87
Cardiac catheterization 4
  enzymes 7
  failure, congestive 68
Cardiomegaly 3
Cardiomyopathy, dilated 5
Catheterization, cardiac 4
  urinary 87
Central cyanosis 10
Cerebral metastases 70
Cervical cancer 71
Charcoal, activated 76
Chest radiograms 88
Chlamydia trachomatis 100
Chromosomes 38
Cirrhosis, liver1
Claudication, intermittent 8
Clostridium tetani 49
Coalworker's pneumoconiosis (CP) 93
Coarctation of the aorta 10
Coeliac disease 31
Colonoscopy 35
Colorectal cancer 35
Congenital aortic stenosis 11
Congestive cardiac failure 68
Constipation 33
Continuous ambulatory peritoneal dialysis 85
Contraceptive, oral 15
Coronary angiography 7
Creatinine, plasma level 82
Crohn's disease 34
Cryptogenic fibrosing alveotitis 93
Cyanosis, central 10
Cyclosporin 84

Cystic fibrosis 32, 90
Dengue fever 53
Depression 78
  postnatal 80
Dermatitis, atopic 21
Dermatological terms 20
Dermatophyte infection 23
Diabetes, dietary advice 24
Diabetes mellitus, non insulin dependent 24
Diabetic ketoacidosis 25
  nephropathy2 5
  retinopathy 24
Dialysis, continuous ambulatory peritoneal 85
Dilated cardiomyopathy 5
Diphtheria 50
Disseminated intravascular coagulation 43
Diverticular disease 36
DNA 38
Double-contrast barium meal 31
Down's syndrome 81
Drowning, management 19
Drug absorption 12
  metabolism 12
Drugs, adverse reactions 15, 17
  antithrombotic 14
  bioavailability 17
  dermatological reactions 20
  modes of action 17
  respiratory complications 89

  routes of administration 16
  routine therapeutic monitoring 17
  serum concentration 12
  side-effects 63, 84
Duchenne muscular dystrophy 38, 64
Duodenal ulceration 30

ECG, T wave 4
ECT 78

Index

EEG 61
Ejection systolic murmurs 3
Encephalitis 48
Endocrine hypertension 29
Endometrial cancer 71
Enuresis, nocturnal 85
Enzyme inducers 13
   inhibitors 13
Enzymes, cardiac 7
Epiglottitis 90
Epileptic fits 63
Epstein-Barr virus 51
Erythema nodosum 20
Ethanol 1

Facial dermatological conditions 21
   palsy, acute 65
   weakness, bilateral 66
Fallot's tetralogy 10
Familial hypophosphataemic
   rickets 102
Family violence 80
Fanconi's syndrome 86
Femoral angioplasty 9
Fibreoptic bronchoscopy 89
Fibrosing alveolitis 93
Fibrosis, progressive massive 93
Filariasis, lymphatic 54
Food additives 68
Foreign body inhalation 90
Fractures, stress 98

Gallstones 58
Gastric adenocarcinoma 31
   surgery 37
   ulceration, benign 30
Gastrointestinal diseases and skin conditions 30
   haemorrhage 30
   histoplasmosis 35
Genital herpes, primary 101
   warts 100
Gingival swelling 75

Glomerular dysfunction 84
Glomerulonephritis 84
Glucocorticoids 14
Glucose-6-phosphate
   dehydrogenase deficiency 41
Gonococcal infection, neonatal 102
Gout 99
Granulocytic leukaemia, chronic 42
Granuloma inguinale 101
Grave's disease 26
Gynaecomastia 28

Haematological abnormalities in
   AIDS 46
   conditions, and dietary
   deficiencies 40
   conditions, laboratory diagnosis 40
Haemolytic disease of the newborn 41
Haemophilia A 43
Haemorrhage, gastrointestinal 30
Heart failure, acute 5
Hepatic amoebiasis 57
   ascites 58
Hepatitis, chronic 57
Hepatitis E 56
Hepatocellular carcinoma 59
Herpes encephalitis 51
   primary genital 101
   simplex proctitis 36
Histoplasmosis, gastrointestinal 35
HIV 45
   antibody test 45
   transmission 45
HLA-DR3, related disorders 44
Hodgkin's disease 73
Hormone, parathyroid 27, 103
Human immunodeficiency virus 45
Huntington's disease 39
Hydatid disease 53
Hypercalcaemia, malignant 69
Hypertension 8

and drugs 8
endocrine 29
portal 59
Hyperthyroidism 26
Hypothyroidism 26

Idiopathic Parkinsonism 65
Imaging, magnetic resonance 98
Immune response, depressed 44
Immunity, active 48
Inappropriate antidiuresis 27
Infarction, myocardial 3, 6, 7
Inheritance of renal disorders 85
Intermittent claudication 8
Interventricular septum, rupture 6
Intestinal schistosomiasis 54
Intracranial aneurysms 63
Intravenous urogram 82
Iron metabolism 40
Irritable bowel syndrome 34
Ischaemic bowel disease 36

Jaundice, prehepatic 57

Kaposi's sarcoma 46
Ketoacidosis, diabetic 25
Kwashiorkor 68

Lactose intolerance 32
Late dumping syndrome3 6
Lavage, bronchoalveolar 89
Leprosy 55
Leptospirosis 55
Leukaemia, acute 42
    acute lymphoblastic 41
    chronic granulocytic 42
    chronic lymphocytic 42
Lithium 79
    adverse effects 79
    poisoning, acute 77
Liver and biliary tract 56
    cirrhosis 1
    disease and protozoa 56

metabolism 56
Loiasis 54
Lumbar puncture 62
Lung cancer 94
    transplantation 95
Lyme disease 52
Lymphadenopathy, persistent generalised 46
Lymphatic filariasis 54
Lymphoblastic leukaemia, acute 41
Lymphocytic leukaemia, chronic 42
Lymphogranuloma verereum 101

Magnetic resonance imaging 98
Malabsorption, post-infective 32
Malaria 53
Malignancy, childhood 74
Marasmus 67
Measles 51
Mechanical ventilation 94
Mediastinal masses 94
Meningiomas 63
Meningitis, meningococcal 48
Meningococcal meningitis 48
Menopause 29
Metabolism, liver 56
Metastases, cerebral 70
Migraine 61
Mitral regurgitation 11
Monoarthritis 99
Morphine 19
Motor neurone disease 65
Mouth, dry 75
    pigmented mucosal lesions 75
Multiple myeloma 72, 73
Multiple sclerosis 62
Muscle groups 61
Myelodysplastic disorders 43
Myeloma, multiple 72, 73
Myocardial infarction 3, 6, 7

Nail signs 22
Necrosis 69

acute tubular 85
Neoplasia, paediatric 73
Nephropathy, diabetic 25
Nerve supply to muscles 61
Neutropenia 70
Nitrates 6
Nocturnal enuresis 85
Non-steroidal anti-inflammatory drugs 98
NSAIDs 98
Nutrition 67

Obstructive pulmonary disease 91
Occupational asthma 91
Oesophageal varices, treatment 58
Onchocerciasis 54
Oral cancer 75
   contraceptive steroids 15
Osteoarthritis 96
Osteomalacia 102
Ovarian cancer 72
Ovary, polycystic 28
Overdoses and antidotes 76

Palpitations 4
Pancreatic cancer 32
Pancreatitis, acute 33
Papillary thyroid carcinoma 26
Parathyroid hormone 27, 103
Parkinsonism, idiopathic 65
PCP 46
Pelvic inflammatory disease (PID) 101
Pericarditis, acute 9
Pericardial effusion 9
Phenylketonuria, classical 39
Plague 55
Plasma creatinine 82
   urea 82
Pleural effusion 88
   fluid, cytology 95
Pneumocystis carinii 92
   pneumonia 46

Pneumonia 92
Poisoning 77
   acute 76
   acute lithium 77
Polio, vaccination 52
Polyarteritis nodosa 60
Polycystic ovary syndrome 28
Portal hypertension 59
Post-infective malabsorption 32
Postnatal depression 80
Pre-eclampsia 83
Pregnancy 83
   skin conditions 21
Prehepatic jaundice 57
Primary biliary cirrhosis 58
Primary genital herpes 101
Progressive massive fibrosis 93
Prostatic cancer 72
Protozoa, and liver disease 56
Pruritus 22
Pseudogout 97
Psoriasis 20
Puberty, delayed 28
Puerperal psychosis 80
Pulmonary disease, obstructive 91
   sarcoidosis 93
PUO 48
Pyridostigmine 64

Rabies 52
Radiotherapy 69
Receptors 13
Red cell destruction 40
Regurgitation, aortic 11
   mitral 11
Reiter's syndrome 97
Renal biopsy, percutaneous 83
   cell carcinoma 87
   ultrasound 82
Respiratory diseases 88
   distress syndrome, adult 18, 94
Retinopathy, diabetic 24

Index

Rheumatoid arthritis, extra-articular
    features 96
    factors 96
Rickets, familial
    hypophosphataemic 102
Rifampicin 92

Sarcoidosis, pulmonary 93
Schistosomiasis, intestinal 54
Schizophrenia 78
Scleroderma 60
Sepsis 18
    life threatening 18
Septal lines on chest radiograms 88
Serum drug concentration 12
Short bowel syndrome 33
Skin conditions and gastrointestinal
    diseases 30
    conditions in pregnancy 21
    lesions 22
Solvent abuse 80
Stenosis, congenital aortic 11
Steroids, oral contraceptive 15
Stomas 35
Stress fractures 98
Stridor, acute 90
Stroke 64
Substance abuse, volatile 2
Superior vena cava, obstruction 70
Swelling, gingival 75
Syndrome of inappropriate
    antidiuresis 27
Syphillis, tertiary 100
Systemic amyloidosis 60
Systemic lupus erythematosus 60
Systolic murmurs, ejection 3
Tertiary syphillis 100
Testosterone 28
Tetralogy of Fallot 10
Theophylline 14
    metabolism 91
    poisoning 77

Thyroid carcinoma 26
TLCO 89
Toxoplasmosis 49
Transplantation, lung 95
Tricyclic antidepressants 79
Tuberous sclerosis, skin lesions 21
Tubular necrosis, acute 85
Typhoid fever 49
Typhus 53

Ulceration, benign gastric 30
    duodenal 30
Ulcerative colitis 34
Ultrasound, renal 82
Unconjugated
    hyperbilirubinaemia 57
Urate stones 86
Urea, plasma level 82
Urinary catheterization 87
    tract infection 86
    tract infection, childhood 86
Urogram, intravenous 82

Valvotomy, aortic 11
Vasodilators, in heart failure 5
Vasopressin 27
Vena cava, superior 70
Ventilation, mechanical 18, 94
Ventricular aneurysms, left 6
    fibrillation 19
    septal defects 10
    tachycardia 19
Violence in the family 80
Viral infections in
    immunocompromised 44
Volatile substance abuse 2
Warts, genital 100
Wilson's disease 39

Yersinia entercolitis 49

Zidovudine, treatment of AIDS 47

PASTEST MEDICAL PUBLICATIONS

The following books, published by PasTest, contain useful revision material for doctors studying for the Royal College of Physicians MRCP Part 1 examination and for other medical examinations containing Multiple Choice Questions.

MRCP Part 1 MCQ Revision Book (3rd edition) *P Kalra*

MRCP Part 1 Practice Exams *P Ackrill*

MRCP Part 1 MCQs with Individual Subject Summaries *P O'Neill*

Explanations to the Royal College of Physicians MRCP(UK) Part 1 Papers (Feb, June, Oct 1990) *H Beynon & C Ross*

Medicine International MCQs Book 3

Oxford Textbook of Medicine MCQs (2nd edition)

MRCP Part 1 MCQ Pocket Books
Book 1:   Cardiology and Respiratory Medicine
Book 2:   Neurology and Psychiatry
Book 3:   Gastroenterology, Endocrinology and Renal Medicine
Book 4:   Haematology, Infectious Diseases and Rheumatology

PasTest Practice Exams and Revision Books are also available for:
MRCP Part 2 General Medicine   DRCOG
MRCP Part 2 Clinical   DCH
MRCP Part 2 Paediatrics   FRCS
MRCGP   FRCA
MRCOG   PLAB

PASTEST INTENSIVE COURSES

PasTest intensive revision courses for many of the above examinations are available. Courses are run before each examination at venues in London and Manchester. All courses offer top quality revision materials and teaching.

For a full catalogue of current titles, courses and prices please contact:
PasTest, Freepost, Knutsford, Cheshire, WA16 7BR
Tel 01565 755226 Fax 01565 650264

16th Jan 5.30pm Dr Herzen
Gl cent L2